ACTIVITIES THERAPY

ACTIVITIES THERAPY

Anne Cronin Mosey, O.T.R., Ph.D., F.A.O.T.A.

Associate Professor
and
Program Director
Occupational Therapy Curriculum
School of Education
New York University

Raven Press, Publishers · New York

Made in the United States of America

International Standard Book Number 0–911216–41–3
Library of Congress Catalog Card Number 73–79286

Fourth Printing, January 1978
Fifth Printing, July 1979
Sixth Printing, September 1980
Seventh Printing, January 1982
Eighth Printing, August 1983

PREFACE

Activities therapy is a relatively new term in the constantly changing jargon of psychiatry. It is used in a limited way to refer to an administrative unit in a psychiatric treatment facility and in a broader sense to refer to a type of treatment. The staff in an activities therapy department usually consists of some mixture of professionally educated people such as art therapists, dance therapists, music therapists, occupational therapists, and recreational therapists, people with particular skills in the arts or crafts, and people who simply have the desire and ability to work with psychiatric patients.

But this book is about activities therapy as a type of treatment—a way of helping people become more active participants in the life of their community.

It is about the use of work-oriented, recreational, and creative-expressive activities as a means of enhancing psychosocial functioning. Activities therapy is not seen as the private domain of people in an activities therapy department but rather as an orientation to treatment which all mental health workers are invited to investigate.

Although activities therapy is a new term, the ideas basic to activities therapy have been around for some time. One of these ideas comes from the concept of therapeutic community or milieu therapy. This type of treatment uses the everyday interactions between patients and staff members and the problems inherent in people living and being together as a way of helping patients acquire skills for independent living. Another idea basic to activities therapy is that the dynamics of group interaction can be used to foster change. The support and demands of a cohesive group often help a patient learn to think, feel, and act in a manner that is more satisfying to himself and others. Activities therapy is based on the idea that psychosocial dysfunction is, at least in part, simply not having learned to function in the wider community. Given this assumption, activities therapy makes use of current knowledge about the teaching-learning proc-

v

ess to develop needed skills in interacting and doing. Finally, activities therapy makes considerable use of the ideas that underlie the action-oriented therapies (i.e., art therapy, therapeutic recreation, occupational therapy, etc.). These therapies use a variety of activities as the vehicle for developing more satisfactory ways of meeting the needs of self and others. The informed reader, therefore, will not find anything new or startling in this book. It is simply an attempt to give some form and shape to these diverse ideas.

Activities therapy, as discussed here, focuses on the treatment of adult psychiatric patients. It may, however, be useful in two other situations. With some modifications, activities therapy may be used in the treatment of emotionally disturbed children. Learning through doing, which is basic to activities therapy, is a natural way for children to acquire knowledge and skills. Again, with some modification, activities therapy may be a useful device for helping the socially disadvantaged. Its orientation, for example, to the development of work habits and satisfactory use of leisure time speaks to some of the real problems in community participation experienced by the socially disadvantaged.

This book is addressed both to students who are preparing to work with psychiatric patients and to those who, with minimal preparation, find themselves working in an activities therapy department. It is important to remember, however, that this book is only an introduction; it is intended to be a supplement to other literature utilized by the various professional preparation curriculums and in-service educational programs. This book is also addressed to the experienced activities therapist, and as such attempts to articulate a meaningful and useful frame of reference for activities therapy, Finally, this book may be of interest to other members of the psychiatric team who would like a clue about what all those activities therapy people are doing.

Table of Contents

CHAPTER 1

INTRODUCTION

What is activities therapy? Activities therapy is stopping a basketball game to help Peter figure out why he has a sudden urge to leave the game, it is Linda testing her capacity to give help through volunteer work in a local nursery school, it is Marsha learning how to budget her welfare money, and it is Jerome practicing cooperation through participation in a rhythm band group. Activities therapy uses immediate, action-oriented interactions to help people who have been designated as "mentally ill" to learn to live in and be a part of their community; it is a method of helping people who are unable to cope with the stresses of daily life.

Mental illness, or psychosocial dysfunction, is defined by an activities therapist as the inability to meet one's needs in a manner that is satisfying to oneself and not detrimental to the need satisfaction of others. The inability to gain need gratification is assumed to be located in the individual as opposed to the environment. Thus, a man who continues to live in an undesirable apartment because he is afraid to look for a more suitable one is considered to be in a state of psychosocial dysfunction. On the other hand, a man who continues to live in an undesirable apartment because there are no suitable apartments available which he can afford to rent is not thought of as being in a state of dysfunction. Activities therapy is based on the assumption that psychosocial dysfunction is the lack of one or more of the following:

> The ability to plan and carry out a task.
> The capacity to interact comfortably in a group.
> The ability to identify and satisfy needs.
> The ability to express emotions in an acceptable manner.
> A more or less accurate perception of the self, the human and non-human environment, and one's relationship to the environment.

1

A value system that allows the individual to satisfy his needs
without infringing on the rights of others.
Skill in carrying out required activities of daily living.
The ability to work at a relatively satisfying job.
Enjoyment of avocational pursuits and recreational activities.
The ability to interact comfortably in family and friendship rela-
tionships.

As a method of treatment, activities therapy is a here-and-now, action-
oriented process which typically involves learning through doing. Activities are used to provide familiar life situations in which participants are
assisted in identifying faulty patterns of behavior and the ideas, feelings,
and values that support these faulty patterns. In turn, participants are
helped to develop more effective ways of acting. For example, Molly
participated in a cooking group only when she was able to take full
responsibility for a specific task, whether shopping, setting the table, or
making the dessert. When this pattern was recognized by one of the other
group members, he began to ask Molly about it. With considerable help
from the group, Molly recognized that sharing a task meant to her that
she would not receive recognition for what she had done. The group then
began to help Molly learn how to get recognition through participating
in a shared task. Activities are also used to develop specific skills. For
example, a group of married women complained of feeling excessively
dependent on their husbands. It was discovered that one reason for this
dependency was an inability to make simple household repairs. At their
request, one of the maintenance men in the treatment center agreed to
teach the women such skills as how to change a fuse, repair a broken
electrical cord, replace a faucet washer, and hang shelving.

These two aspects of activities therapy—greater understanding of self
and development of skills—are interdependent. That is, one area is not
seen as being more important than the other, nor is deficit in one area
viewed as the cause of deficit in the other area. The therapist is concerned
with both areas throughout the entire treatment process. A division between understanding of self and development of skills is made only to
clarify what occurs in activities therapy. As we shall see later, there is
considerable overlap between these areas.

In the actual treatment setting, some treatment situations may be structured to enhance self-understanding while other situations may be de-

signed to enhance skill development. For example, a mural painting group may be used to explore needs and emotions, while a simple assembly-line work operation may be designed to develop work habits. However, if an opportunity arises in either group to facilitate learning in the area not of primary concern, the therapist usually takes advantage of the opportunity. For example, Paul was an active member of the mural group, but his general appearance was so dirty and unkempt that it was offensive to other group members. The group discussed this with Paul, and he agreed to try to do something about his grooming. Group members took responsibility for checking Paul's appearance at the beginning of each session and complimenting him for every improvement.

Activities therapy may occur in a group or in a one-to-one situation. An example of group activities therapy has been given above. One example of individual activities therapy is Joan meeting regularly with a therapist to correct a faulty body image. Joan felt that her body was very large when in fact she was of average height and rather slender. One technique used was to have Joan experience her body in a variety of different-sized spaces. This involved such activities as crawling under furniture, going into broom closets and lockers, sitting and standing in enclosures she had made with large blocks, and experimenting with different-sized playground equipment.

The decision of whether group or individual activities therapy should be used depends on the needs of the individual patient. Pragmatically, if the setting has no groups designed to deal with a patient's particular problem, he is usually helped in a one-to-one treatment situation.

Activities therapy may involve discussion only, with no task being done during the meetings. Rather, attention is focused on a specific task that all group members share. They may be currently attempting to engage in the task in the wider community or they may anticipate undertaking the task in the immediate future. The group discusses how to carry out the task and problems that have been or may be encountered. Role playing is often used to facilitate learning. Some examples are discussion groups concerned with how to apply for a job, utilize leisure time, find an apartment, care for preschool children, and manage a household.

The above brief introduction to activities therapy may have raised some question in the reader's mind. Perhaps a few definitions would be helpful before we proceed. First, the term *treatment* is here conceived as being a planned, collaborative interaction between the therapist, the patient, and, at times, the nonhuman environment, directed toward the development of skills for community living. *Planned and collaborative interaction* refers to the idea that the therapist and patient have clearly identified what changes they hope to bring about and what each of them is going to do to attain these previously set goals. For example, a patient and therapist may have decided that one of the patient's problems is that he cannot express his anger. The therapist, using his knowledge of how people can learn to express anger, designs an appropriate learning situation. The patient is told what is expected of him when he is involved in the learning situation, and what the therapist's role will be. Treatment is a partnership; the patient and therapist work together.

The term *nonhuman environment* refers to all aspects of the external environment that are not human. It includes natural objects such as animals, clouds, plants, and water as well as man-made objects such as buildings, household articles, musical instruments, toys, and machinery. In treatment we are concerned with the nonhuman environment for two reasons. Patients are helped to learn how to manipulate and master the nonhuman environment. For example, patients may be taught how to cook, play tennis, follow a subway map, or fill out job-application forms. The nonhuman environment is also used to help patients acquire greater self-understanding and more satisfying interpersonal relationships. Use of the nonhuman environment is secondary in this case in that it is a means for learning something else. For example, finger painting may be used to help patients identify their needs or to express emotions, or planning and giving a party may be used to help patients learn how to work with others.

Perhaps of more concern to the reader is the previous discussion of psychosocial dysfunction as lack of the knowledge, skills, and values needed for community living. The reader may be more accustomed to thinking of psychosocial dysfunction as "unconscious conflict," and may assume that a person will be able to function in the community once he has resolved his unconscious conflicts. Further, it is often thought that the only valid form of treatment is individual or group verbal psychotherapy. Any other kind of treatment is seen as being second best or to be used only when the patient does not seem able to participate in verbal psychotherapy. There are many theories regarding the nature and cause of psychosocial dysfunction. But no theory has been found to be totally acceptable when subjected to scientific study. Similarly, there are many different ideas about what is the best kind of treatment. It is very difficult to evaluate the effects of treatment. However, at the present time, no one is able to say that one form of treatment is better than another kind of treatment. There is so much that is not known about psychosocial dysfunction; it is a secret that as of now remains unresolved.

Activities therapy is based on the idea that psychosocial dysfunction is learned maladaptive behavior. The individual has developed patterns of behavior that are ineffective in coping with the demands of daily life. It is believed that these faulty patterns of behavior can be unlearned and replaced by other, more effective patterns. This does not mean that activities therapy is not concerned about the ideas, feelings, and values that influence behavior. Identifying one's ideas about himself and others and one's feelings and values is an important part of activities therapy. Treatment does involve examination of these areas; it is concerned with helping a person make "internal" changes as well as behavioral changes. The term "unconscious conflict" is not used in this book because it is too vague. It is too often assigned a magical, mysterious quality that is not particularly useful in thinking about psychosocial dysfunction.

One way in which activities therapy differs from some of the more traditional therapies is in its emphasis on the present. How the patient came to be in a state of psychosocial dysfunction is of little concern. There is no attempt to gather information about events that took place in the distant past. The activities therapist does not believe that a person must know what past events caused him to be in a state of psychosocial dysfunction before any change is possible. The therapist is concerned primarily with where the patient is right now and the nature of his present life situation. Treatment is directed toward the development of knowledge, skills, and values that the patient will need in the future.

A few words about therapeutic drugs and their relation to the ideas about psychosocial dysfunction that are basic to activities therapy are appropriate here. There are several drugs that appear to be effective in minimizing thought disorders, anxiety, depression, and hyperactivity. Therapeutic drugs are usually given to correct a biochemical imbalance, but this is not the case with the psychoactive drugs being discussed here. No chemical imbalance has been found in individuals for whom these drugs are prescribed. They are prescribed because they have been found to be effective for at least some people. How and why these drugs work is, as of now, still unknown. Patients who receive drugs sometimes show such marked improvement that no other type of treatment is needed.

Other patients improve somewhat but need additional help in learning how to function in the community. A few patients seem unaffected by even massive doses of psychoactive drugs. Given all of the unknowns, psychosocial dysfunction could be caused by either chemical imbalance or interaction in an environment that did not allow for the learning of adequate skills for community living or both. Pragmatically, about all that can be said at this point is that if treatment through the use of therapeutic drugs alone is effective—great. If it is not effective, let us try something else.

In summary, activities therapy is based on the assumption that psychosocial dysfunction is a lack of understanding of the self or the inability to participate in the varied and complex tasks of everyday life or both. As a treatment process, activities therapy is here and now, action-oriented, and involves learning through doing. Emphasis is on mastery of the nonhuman environment, and nonhuman objects are utilized in activities designed to enhance self-awareness and interpersonal relationships. The activities used in activities therapy are similar to typical life experiences of the community. Activities therapy is concerned with growth through action.

SUGGESTED READING

Becker, Ernest. *The Revolution in Psychiatry.* New York: The Free Press of Glencoe, 1964.

Cumming, J., and Cumming, E. *Ego and Milieu.* New York: Atherton Press, 1966.

Edelson, Marshall. *Ego Psychology, Group Dynamics, and the Therapeutic Community.* New York: Grune & Stratton, 1964.

Hyde, Robert. *Milieu Rehabilitation.* Providence, R.I.: Butler Health Center, 1967.

Jones, Maxwell. *Social Psychiatry in Practice.* London: Penguin Books, 1968.

London, Perry. *The Modes and Morals of Psycho-Therapy.* New York: Holt, Rinehart & Winston, 1964.

Rogers, C., and Stevens, Barry. *Person to Person.* New York: Pocket Books, 1971.

Searles, Harold. *The Nonhuman Environment.* New York: International Universities Press, 1960.

CHAPTER 2

FACETS OF MAN

Before she can help another person, a therapist must understand what a well-integrated, happy, and productive person is able to do. Using this understanding, the therapist can then assist a patient in determining what his present assets are and what additional knowledge, skill, and attitudes he may need to acquire. The purpose of this chapter is to provide some basic information about the multiple abilities and talents that enable a person to be an active participant in the life of his community.

People are very complicated: They think, feel, and act in a variety of situations and on many different levels, and their thinking, feeling, and acting are highly complex and interrelated. In order to talk about man, it is first necessary to break up his extremely complicated nature into manageable units. In doing this here, we shall speak of the many "facets" of man. The term *facets* was chosen to draw an analogy between the nature of man and a cut gem. It is the complementary interplay of the small, polished, plane surfaces of a precious stone that gives it beauty. A single facet of a cut gem, considered in isolation, tends to be a bit sterile and gives only a minuscule idea of what the whole could or will be. Similarly, the facets of man that we shall discuss here may appear to be somewhat disconnected and lacking in depth. However, the reader is asked to think of these separate areas as facets which, when interrelated and viewed together, will reflect the beauty of man.

BASIC SKILLS

Task skills and group-interaction skills are referred to as *basic* skills because a person cannot function in the community if he is unable to perform simple activities and to interact with other people. They are also referred to as basic because they are fundamental to many of the other things one must do to satisfy needs and contribute to the community.

7

Task Skills

Man is action-oriented: Anyone who stays in bed all day, or just sits in a chair for hours on end doing nothing, is considered "different" at least. One must do, act, perform in order to be considered normal. This is not to say that moments of reverie and quiet relaxation are not a normal part of life, but that the pleasure derived from such experiences usually grows out of past activity or anticipated activity.

It is somewhat difficult to talk about task skills, since the question of what level of skill is being discussed is often raised. For our purpose, determining level of skill will involve comparison. Thus, in looking at another individual's task skills, one asks himself, "Is this person able to do the kinds of things that another person of similar age and background is able to do?"

Task skills here include the following:

> A fairly normal rate of performance.
> Appropriate use of tools and materials.
> Willingness to engage in doing tasks.
> Sustained interest in a task.
> The ability to follow demonstrated, oral, and written directions.
> An acceptable level of neatness.
> Appropriate attention to detail.
> The ability to solve problems that arise in performing a task.
> The ability to organize tasks in a logical manner.

In the normal course of development, many task skills are learned through play. This is an ideal situation for learning task skills because, in true play, failure is unimportant, there is minimal pressure, and there is much time for experimentation. It is more difficult to acquire task skills when there is a high demand for successful performance.

Group-Interaction Skills

Group-interaction skill is the ability to be a productive member of a variety of small groups. Any activity that is shared with more than one other person involves the use of group-interaction skills. The ability to function in a group seems to develop in a sequential pattern in the normal development process. Subskills are acquired in a step-by-step manner until the individual is able to function effectively in a fairly complex and demanding group situation.

The stages of development of group-interaction skills appear to be as follows:

The Ability to Participate in a Parallel Group. A parallel group is characterized by individuals working or playing in the presence of others, by minimal sharing of tasks, and by mutual stimulation. Examples of the latter are making other people laugh, imitation, tentative testing of the effects of one's behavior on others, and casual conversation.

The Ability to Participate in a Project Group. A project group is characterized by membership involvement in short-term tasks that require some sharing or interaction. The interaction may be cooperative or competitive in nature. The task is the only thing that is shared; there is little interaction other than that necessary to perform the task.

The Ability to Participate in an Egocentric-Cooperative Group. Egocentric-cooperative groups are characterized by group members deciding on relatively long-term activites and carrying them through to completion. The joint interaction is based on a mutual belief that individual rights will be respected only through respect for the rights of others. Individuals in this type of group are able to meet each other's esteem needs (see p. 13), but they are not yet able to meet each other's love and safety needs (see p. 12).

The Ability to Participate in a Cooperative Group. A cooperative group is usually made up of individuals who have common interests, concerns, and values. The activity is relatively unimportant in this type of group; the members may come together simply to be together. There is a sense of mutuality and warm involvement in the group.

The Ability to Participate in a Mature Group. A mature group is usually made up of people with different backgrounds, ages, interests, and ideas. Members are able to take a variety of roles as the need for various roles arises in the group. There is a good balance between task accomplishment and satisfaction of group members' needs.

Many people do not attain a high level of group-interaction skill and still manage to function in the community. A considerable number of work and recreational situations, however, require at least the ability to interact in an egocentric-cooperative group. Lack of this ability cuts a person off from many of the need-satisfying and rewarding experiences that are available in the community.

The development of group-interaction skill occurs through participation in the various types of groups outlined above. These groups are usually readily available during childhood and adolescence. They can be found arising spontaneously on the playground, in school, and in recreational facilities. More structured group learning experiences are also available in the school situation, as well as in camps, church clubs, sports teams, and special interest groups.

THE PRIVATE SELF

Cognitive system, needs, emotions, and values are here referred to as the private self because they are essentially located within the individual. We cannot see or experience these aspects of another person directly. We can only make educated guesses about another person's private self through observation of his behavior or from what he tells us.

Cognitive System

Cognitive system refers to what a person knows and thinks about himself, other people, and the world around him. Included in the cognitive system is factual knowledge (one should cross the street on a green light) and beliefs or ideas (all men are created equal). Of primary importance is what an individual thinks of himself as a person. This group of ideas is sometimes referred to as *self-concept*. Self-concept usually includes ideas about what one looks like, what kind of person one is, and what one is able to do and not able to do. Of equal importance is an individual's ideas about other people—what they are like and how they are likely to respond? Knowledge about how things work and what one should do in various situations is also a significant part of the cognitive system.

Two processes influence how an individual thinks: conceptualization and identification of relationships. Conceptualization is the process of categorizing or placing things into groups. For example, through repeated experiences a child learns the difference between feeling hungry and feeling thirsty and the difference between a ball and a toy car. Each of these feelings and objects is seen as having something in common that makes it different from everything else. Thus, they are placed in separate categories. Conceptualization is evident even before a child learns to talk; after a certain age he will not passively take whatever is offered but will, for example, refuse to eat his cereal when he wants a drink of juice. Similarly, when a young child is given a ball, he tends to throw it rather than run it along the table as if it were a toy car. *Labeling* is giving a name to a category. Most of the words we use are labels for some class of events, nonhuman objects, people, actions, and the like.

The second process is identification of relationships: what goes with what, what causes something to happen, sequences of events, and so forth. It is through knowledge of numerous relationships that we come to know how to influence people and manipulate things. We learn, for example, that certain types of behavior will earn praise in one situation and be laughed at in another situation. We learn that a car will not run if the engine is flooded.

The knowledge a person has acquired may be accurate or inaccurate, sufficient or insufficient, conscious or unconscious. Examples of inaccurate knowledge are Philip labeling himself homosexual when there is no evidence this is true or Martha believing that other people can read her thoughts. Insufficient knowledge is demonstrated by Anne's inability to make change from a five-dollar bill and by William when he says he does not know what other people think of him. Michael's knowledge about his emotions is unconscious when he honestly says he does not feel anger but continues to act in a very angry manner. Beth, an intelligent and charming girl, states that she wants to get married but finds considerable fault with any likely candidate, because she has the unconscious belief that men are interested only in her physical attractions.

As the latter example indicates, much of a person's unconscious knowledge is inaccurate. However, this is not always the case. Unconscious knowledge of group process is evident in an individual who functions well in a group but is unable to talk about what he is doing. People guide their actions by using both unconscious knowledge and conscious knowledge. Accurate unconscious knowledge does not usually interfere with adequate functioning. Inaccurate unconscious knowledge often does interfere.

An individual is considered to have sufficient, accurate, conscious knowledge when he is aware of his needs, emotions, and values, when he has ideas about himself and others that are shared by most other people, when he knows his capacities and limitations, and when he is knowledgeable about what effect his behavior has on others and how other people affect him. A fully functioning individual must know enough about the human and nonhuman environment to be able to interact with it in a comfortable manner.

Needs

All people have a variety of basic human needs, which they attempt to satisfy in a number of ways. These needs, as they are discussed here, are considered to be inherent as opposed to learned or acquired. One of the major tasks every individual faces is learning how to meet his needs to the fullest possible extent without harming himself or infringing on the rights of others.

Human needs have been categorized in many different ways. Here we shall combine several classical systems and describe normal human needs as physiological, safety, love and belonging, mastery, esteem, and self-actualization.

Physiological Needs. Physiological needs must be satisfied in order to maintain life. They include the need for air, food, shelter, an optimal amount of sensory stimuli and motor activity, and the release of sexually induced tensions. When there is deprivation of physiological needs, the individual's attention is usually focused almost exclusively on their satisfaction. Other needs become relatively unimportant.

Safety Needs. Safety needs are satisfied through interacting in an environment that is experienced as relatively free of harmful situations. Such an environment is characterized by (a) general agreement about what is right and wrong, (b) predictable responses from others, (c) knowledge regarding what behavior is expected of each individual, (d) recognition of the individual's right to need satisfaction, (e) lack of arbitrary decision making, (f) some degree of change as a consequence of the individual's actions, (g) a limited number of things the individual cannot understand or influence, and (h) freedom from physical harm. People try to avoid situations that they think are unsafe. If most situations are so viewed, the individual becomes very constricted in his interactions. This, in turn, limits the opportunity to gain satisfaction of other needs.

Love and Belonging Needs. Love and belonging needs are satisfied when an individual is accepted by others as being a unique and very special person. The individual must be accepted for himself rather than for something he has done or is doing. In addition, the individual must be recognized as a valuable part of some aggregate of people; he must have a sense of kinship with others.

Mastery Needs. The need to master refers to the desire to explore, understand, and to some extent control oneself, other people, and the nonhuman environment. It is the desire to figure out how things work, to test one's abilities, to match wits with another person. When motivated by mastery needs, an individual engages in an activity for the pleasure he derives from the activity.

Esteem Needs. Esteem needs motivate an individual to engage in an activity in order to receive recognition from others. The activity in and of itself may not be seen as or be pleasurable. The individual desires to receive respect for his actions, for being productive or creative. These needs can be satisfied only if a person has an opportunity to do something that is perceived by others as being worthwhile.

Self-actualization Needs. The need for self-actualization is the need to be oneself—to do something that is of particular importance to oneself. Activities motivated by this need are self-oriented in that recognition or acknowledgement from others is not required for satisfaction. The self-actualization need is different from the need to master in that mastery involves some kind of struggle or contest. In satisfying self-actualization needs there may be struggle, but that is not the point of doing the activity. The poet, for example, may work very hard to write a poem just exactly the way he wants it to be, but that is not why he writes poetry. He writes to satisfy a desire to express his ideas; it is his way of attaining self-actualization.

People meet their needs in a number of different ways. A particular activity may satisfy one need for one person and another need for another person. For example, some people cook because they are hungry (physical need), others because they like the praise they receive from family or friends (esteem need), and still others because they like to cook (self-actualization). Similarly, one person may learn karate to satisfy his need for safety, whereas another person may learn it to gain a sense of mastery of his own body.

One of the major tasks that faces every individual is learning how to meet his own needs in a socially acceptable manner. In order for this to occur, the individual must experience both need satisfaction and an optimal amount of need deprivation. Optimal refers to the degree of need deprivation that allows the individual to be aware that a need is not being satisfied, but not so much deprivation that the person experiences a strong negative emotion. For example, in helping a child develop the ability to satisfy esteem needs, a mother praises her child for doing almost anything when he is very young. Later she requires that he do simple tasks in order to receive her praise. Ideally, the tasks the mother asks the child to perform are ones the child can perform without too much difficulty.

A person must also learn what his needs are. Many people have a vague feeling of frustration because they are not satisfying one or several of their needs. Lack of satisfaction in this case is not due to environmental deprivation or lack of ability on the part of the individual; rather, the person does not know that the need is not being satisfied. For example, many people say they are bored when their real difficulty is that they are not satisfying their need for mastery.

In learning how to satisfy needs, the individual also learns to live with some degree of need deprivation. For example, safety needs are not usually fully met during the first few weeks on a new job. The new worker has to "feel out" the situation, learn what is expected of him, learn the unwritten rules, and discover channels of communication. A person who cannot tolerate this type of need deprivation may leave the job. He may, in fact, never be able to hold a job because he cannot tolerate the initial feeling of insecurity.

The right time and place is also important in learning how to satisfy needs. For example, the student often has to come to realize that his need for love is not going to be met by his instructors. He must seek satisfaction of this need elsewhere. The Sunday painter often takes up this activity because his need for self-actualization cannot be met in his work situation.

Emotions

Emotions are inherent responses to need satisfaction and deprivation. They arise not only from the objective degree of satisfaction and deprivation but are closely related to the person's view of the situation. Emotions are both positive and negative.

The positive emotions are responses to need fulfillment. They are here labeled as satisfaction, joy, liking, and love. Satisfaction is the response to need fulfillment that is considered acceptable by the individual. Joy is the response to an above-average degree of need fulfillment. Liking is the response to a person or thing that is associated with an acceptable degree of need satisfaction. Love is the response to a person or thing that provides a much higher than average degree of need fulfillment. In order for positive emotions to be experienced, the individual must expect that need fulfillment will continue. For example, one rarely feels liking for a person who satisfies love and belonging needs only on rare occasions.

Negative emotions are associated with need deprivation. They are here labeled dissatisfaction, fear, dislike, hatred, anger, and depression. Dissatisfaction is the response to need deprivation. Fear is the response to anticipated loss of need fulfillment, for example, "I'm afraid to speak because I may make a fool of myself." (No distinction is made here between fear and anxiety, because the difference between the two concepts is very vague.) Anger is the response to need deprivation when the individual believes that he has a right to need fulfillment. Dislike and hatred are degrees of a negative feeling about a person or situation seen as need-depriving or potentially depriving. Depression is the response to the loss of a need-fulfilling person, thing, or situation. It occurs when the individual believes there is no substitute for what has been lost. For example, a woman who has no other interests but her children is likely to feel depressed when the children grow up and leave home. A woman with many interests other than her children will probably not become depressed. Guilt, also, is usually considered to be a negative emotion. However, rather than being related to need deprivation, it is the response to an attempt at or actual fulfillment of needs in a manner that is unacceptable to the individual.

As mentioned above, emotional responses are inherent; they are not learned. What is learned is one's ideas about a situation. For example, George feels fearful when he must go to visit in another town. He is afraid that he will get lost; his need for security is threatened. John, on the other hand, knows he may get lost, but he also knows there is always a means of finding the right way. Thus he does not experience fear.

Emotional responses are an internal experience. Emotional expression is the outward manifestation of an emotional response. Emotional expression is learned. An individual is able to express his emotions adequately when the overt manifestations of his emotions are sufficient to inhibit formation of an uncomfortable amount of internal tension and sufficiently controlled so as not to interfere significantly with current or future need fulfillment. Adequate emotional expression is best learned in an environment that accepts all emotions as legitimate. In other words, there must be people around who indicate by word and action that an individual has a right to experience all of the emotions. However, people often act as though some emotions are bad. A person raised in such an environment may not only have difficulty expressing his emotions, he may not even know that he is experiencing a particular emotion. He sees the emotion as so bad that he refuses to acknowledge it. Other elements that are required for learning adequate emotional expression are opportunity for trial-and-error practice and good models for imitation.

The learning of adequate negative emotional expression is closely related to learning how to meet one's own needs. If the individual is required to meet only those aspects of his needs that he is currently capable or almost capable of meeting, emotional responses will not become too intense. If an emotion is too intense, it is more difficult to express it in an acceptable way. Adequate emotional expression is more easily acquired when the emotion is experienced but not to such an intense degree that it is overwhelming to the individual. There is another relationship between emotional expression and learning how to fulfill needs. Frequently the problem is not the learning of adequate emotional expression, but rather learning how to meet needs so that negative emotions are kept to a minimum. Thus, for example, it is often more useful to help a person learn how to deal with whatever people or situations are making him angry than it is to help him learn how to express his anger.

Values

Values are the degree of worth ascribed to a person, thing, activity, or idea. The words right and wrong, good and bad, should and should not are statements of values. Values are seen as being on a continuum: high positive, low positive, low negative, high negative. There is no neutral point on this continuum. It is here assumed that every individual places some value on everything. However, he may not be aware of what value he has placed on a particular thing. The sum total of an individual's values is referred to as his value system or system of values. The tendency to place values is inherent; the particular value assigned to a person, thing, activity, or idea is learned.

Values are acquired in two ways. The first is through direct experience. The individual places negative value on anything he sees as related to his need deprivation and positive value on anything related to his need fulfill-ment. The degree of negative or positive value depends on the degree of deprivation or fulfillment the individual experiences. The second way in which values are acquired is by taking on the value system of another person or group of people. In order for this to occur, the individual must see these others as people who fulfill or are likely to fulfill his needs. In addition, he must believe that taking on this particular value system will lead to continued need fulfillment.

Because of these two ways of acquiring values, an individual may have a value system that is not internally consistent. That is, he may assign both a positive and a negative value to the same thing. For example, George experiences school as interfering with satisfaction of his needs. His parents, whom he still needs for support, assign a high positive value to school. George then comes to view school as both negative and positive. This is referred to as being ambivalent about something. Another source of difficulty is that an individual may grow up in an environment where the value system is not only inconsistent, but where the stated values may not actually be the true values used in the environment. Examples of the first difficulty in our culture can be seen in the ambivalence regarding motherhood, busing, or welfare. An example of the second difficulty is Susan's father preaching honesty while he brings home large quantities of office supplies for his personal use.

An adequate system of values allows an individual to satisfy his needs without interfering with the need satisfaction of others. An inadequate system of values leads to need deprivation for the individual or other people.

THE PUBLIC SELF

Activities of daily living, work, recreation, and intimacy are referred to as aspects of the public self since they are more directly related to interactions with others. These are aspects of an individual that can be observed by another person. They are the point of contact between the self and others. The public self and the private self strongly influence one another. Many needs, for example, are gratified through work and recrea-tion. Ideas about other people affect one's ability to engage in intimate relations.

Activities of Daily Living

Activities of daily living refer to all those *other* things a person must be able to do in order to engage successfully in work, recreation, and intimacy. The list of these activities is essentially endless. However, for convenience, activities of daily living may be divided into three areas: care of the self, communication, and travel. Care of the self includes such things as washing, getting dressed, mending clothes, getting a meal, and budgeting money. Communication involves using the telephone, writing personal letters, getting information, and being able to fill out forms. Travel includes such things as using public transportation, knowing how to read a subway or road map, driving a car, and being able to get a taxi. Competence in activities of daily living allows one to pay attention to "more important" or significant life events. When a person must give considerable attention to the activities of daily living, there is little energy left for dealing with any other part of existence.

What may be an activity of daily living for one person may be work or recreation for another person. Driving a car is work for the taxi driver; it is an activity of daily living for a factory worker who must drive to work; it is recreation for the sports car enthusiast. An individual's orientation also influences how one would describe a particular activity. For example, a housewife may consider getting breakfast every morning for her family as one of her work responsibilities. However, she may see preparing a special meal for company as recreation.

Work

Work is a person's major occupation: It is what an individual does to make money. This is not to say that the only reason people work is to make money, but it is an important factor. Work also can lead to a considerable degree of need satisfaction. A person's occupation often provides a sense of identity, a sense of relationship to the wider community. Although not performed for monetary reward, a homemaker's responsibilities for maintaining a congenial home and child rearing are here considered to be work. Similarly, the work of a student is studying and being able to get along with classmates and teachers.

Our society holds many different attitudes about work, from "work is good in and of itself" to "work is a necessary evil," and from "one should strive to get to the top" to "striving for success is a false goal." The attitudes one has toward work influence how important work is to a given individual; they influence an individual's priorities relative to work. It is difficult to speak of "the right attitude" toward work, that is, what value should be placed on work. There is considerable variation as to what is acceptable in one cultural group as opposed to another cultural group. Perhaps it is sufficient to say at this point that an individual should place enough positive value on work to get a job if he needs to work to support himself.

Aside from attitudes, the ability to work involves certain basic knowledge and skills. These are often referred to as *work habits.* Some examples of work habits are being able to get to work on time and working a full work day, dressing appropriately, being able to accept direction from a work supervisor, taking responsibility for assigned tasks, and being able to get along with one's co-workers. Good work habits are the kinds of things one must be able to do in order to be successful in any job. Other, more specific skills are also required for various types of jobs.

Recreation

There are two aspects to recreation. The first involves those things a person does for fun or relaxation. These might include reading a novel, taking a walk, watching television, going to a party, playing baseball, and swimming. The second aspect of recreation involves community activities. Examples of community activities are doing volunteer work in a hospital or nursing home, participating in politics, tutoring a student, being a Girl Scout leader, organizing a rent strike, and planning a block party.

Recreation has become increasingly important for many people in our society; the work week has become shorter, and an increasing number of persons are retired. More people have more free time to spend in recreational activities. Recreation has also become more important as people receive less need satisfaction from their jobs. One problem frequently encountered is the use of free time—time not devoted to work, activities of daily living, and intimacy. People often engage repeatedly in the same recreational activities long after the activities have ceased to be need satisfying. They complain of boredom and lack of involvement. This problem may be compounded by a lack of recreational facilities in the community. In order for recreational activities to be meaningful, a person must be aware of his needs. Otherwise he tends to do what everyone else is doing; there is a vague feeling of dissatisfaction, the source of which remains unidentified. Ideally, selection of recreational activities is a conscious choice, considered and planned with care. New recreational activities are started on a trial basis, a commitment being made only if the activity is found to be truly need satisfying. Doing something because one thinks one ought to do so is really not recreation.

The division between work and recreation is admittedly vague. For some people, caring for their lawn is definitely work; it is a chore that must be done. For others, the care of a lawn and garden is a source of great pleasure. There are some people who gain so much satisfaction from their work that in many ways they think of it as recreation. Julia Child, for example, seems to derive so much pleasure from her gourmet cooking that one suspects she would not describe her cooking as work.

There are some people who do not appear to engage in any recreational activities. They never seem to relax and enjoy themselves. If they are not engaged in occupational pursuits, they are "working" at something else. Either of two things may be happening in this situation. The individual may derive so much satisfaction from his occupation and other work-like chores that he honestly feels no need for more typical recreational activities. On the other hand, the person may not seem to have any interest in recreational activities. In this case he may not know how to engage in such activities, or he may have placed a high negative value on recreational activities.

Intimacy

Intimacy is that area of human experience that involves a close, sustained relationship with other individuals. Without such relationships an individual often feels lonely and uninvolved in the mainstream of human life. The ability to engage in intimate behavior is a skill that develops over time. Like group-interaction skills, intimacy appears to be acquired in stages. The skills learned at each stage are not lost, but remain a part of the pool of abilities available for use by the individual in appropriate situations. This is true, as we shall see, for all stages except chum relationships.

The stages of development of intimacy are as follows.

Casual Friendships. Being able to form casual friendships includes the capacity to reach out and make friends. It is the ability to experience pleasure in being with other people, whether doing things together or simply talking. There is a sense of sharing in a casual friendship, of having common interests and values. The word *casual* is used here to indicate that this type of friendship is not particularly intense. For example, it could be characterized by the statement, "I like her and enjoy her company; I would miss her if she left town tomorrow, but there are other people I like being with just as much." Casual friendships provide mutual need satisfaction, but the satisfaction is not considered to be central in one's life experience.

Chum Relationships. Chum relationships usually develop in preadolescents with one or two other persons of the same age and sex. This is an extremely intense relationship in which the individuals want to be together as often as possible. There is a secrecy about the relationship. Others are excluded and seen as interfering. One partner experiences jealousy and hurt if he feels the other partner is paying too much attention to someone else. In a mutual chum relationship, the individuals trust each other implicitly and share their more intimate thoughts and ideas. The needs of one's partner are seen as being as important as one's own needs.

Once a person has experienced one or two chum relationships, he rarely returns to this intense, total involvement with another person. His relationships, although very close, do not have the components of jealousy and the need to be together at all times. Chum relationships seem to provide an opportunity to experiment with satisfying another person's need for love and to develop empathy and compassion.

Love Relationships. Love relationships are mutually need satisfying. They are sustained over a long period of time despite occasional conflicts and differences of opinion. The partners are willing to make sacrifices for each other. Love relationships differ from chum relationships in that each partner feels free to participate in other love and friendship relationships. Love relationships are quite different from casual friendships. People who love each other experience a great sense of loss when the relationship is disrupted. There is a feeling that the partner cannot be replaced by another person. Loss of a loved one leaves a "hole" in one's existence. It is only after a period of adjustment that one can even think about finding someone else to take the place of the loved partner. As the term "love relationship" is used here, it describes not only ideal sexual relationships but also the relationships between close friends.

Nurturing Relationships. A nurturing relationship is one in which one partner helps the other to grow toward his unique potential. The nurturing partner is able to satisfy the needs of the other partner without demanding similar need satisfaction in return. For example, a mother satisfies her child's safety needs, but she does not expect the child to satisfy her safety needs. The nurturing partner gives time, energy, and unconditional love freely. In a good nurturing relationship growth is encouraged, with general goals in mind, but there is no idea of molding the individual to become a specific type of person. The nurturing partner is able to give up his nurturing relationship when the nurtured partner is ready to continue growing on his own. Nurturing relationships are found not only between parent and child but also between teacher and pupil, therapist and patient, skilled worker and neophyte, and so forth.

SUMMARY

This chapter has identified facets of man that appear to be important for a person's full and satisfying participation in the life of the community. It has attempted to outline what a person needs to know and the things he should be able to do in order to be a functioning person. The reader may feel that important areas have not been covered or that some of the facets outlined are of minor importance. This is to be encouraged. The purpose of the chapter is to emphasize that the activities therapist must have some framework for assessing a patient's problem areas. The specific framework used is not as important as the concept of having some framework as the basis for thinking about one's work as a helping person.

SUGGESTED READING

Arieti, Silvano. *The Intrapsychic Self.* New York: Basic Books, 1967.

Black, Max. *The Importance of Language.* Ithaca: Cornell University Press, 1962.

Borow, Heney. *Man in a World of Work.* Boston: Houghton Mifflin Company, 1964.

Brantley, H., and Sessoms, D. *Recreation: Issues and Perspectives.* Columbia, S.C.: Wing Publications, 1969.

Erikson, Erik. *Childhood and Society.* New York: W. W. Norton, 1950.

Friedenberg, Edger. *Coming of Age in America.* New York: Random House, 1963.

Gorlow, L., and Katkunsky, R. *Readings in the Psychology of Adjustment.* New York: McGraw-Hill Book Company, 1968.

Group for the Advancement of Psychiatry, Committee on Adolescence. *Normal Adolescence: Its Dynamics and Impact.* New York: Charles Scribner's Sons, 1968.

Hoffman, Adeline. *Daily Needs and Interests of Older People.* Springfield, Ill.: Charles C Thomas, 1970.

Kraus, Richard. *Recreation and Leisure in Modern Times.* New York: Appleton-Century-Crofts, 1971.

Maslow, Abraham. *Towards a Psychology of Being.* Princeton, N.J.: D. Van Nostrand Company, 1962.

Neugarten, Bernice. *Personality in Middle and Late Life.* Chicago: University of Chicago Press, 1968.

Pearce, J., and Newton, S. *The Conditions of Human Growth.* New York: Citadel Press, 1963.

Super, Donald. *The Psychology of Careers.* New York: Harper & Row, 1957.

Thomson, Robert. *The Psychology of Thinking.* Baltimore: Penguin Books, 1959.

White, Robert. "Competence and the Growth of Personality," in J. Masserman (Ed.), *The Ego.* New York: Grune & Stratton, 1967.

CHAPTER 3

THE TEACHING-LEARNING PROCESS

The last chapter discussed some ideas about man and the kinds of things a person needs to learn in order to participate in the life of the community. This necessary learning usually takes place in the normal course of growing up, and most people tend to be relatively unaware of the learning process. For a person in a state of psychosocial dysfunction, however, all of this learning did not occur. Something went astray, so that the individual did not acquire the knowledge, skills, and values that he needed. Treatment for such individuals is directed toward learning or development of necessary living skills. Some characteristics of the environment that facilitate learning were mentioned in the last chapter. However, the activities therapist needs additional information about the teaching-learning process to design truly adequate learning experiences for patients. This chapter, therefore, will examine the teaching-learning process in more detail.

DEFINITION OF THE TEACHING-LEARNING PROCESS

Learning is a process that we can perceive only through change in an individual's verbal or nonverbal behavior. We say that a person has learned something when he does something one day that he was unable to do the day before, or that he does something differently from the way he did it the day before. The changes in behavior that occur as a result of the use of drugs, some chemical deficit of the body or chemical imbalance, and of brain damage are not considered to be learning.

Learning takes place within a person. A teacher can only design a situation that he believes will enhance or facilitate learning; the learner does the actual learning. It is very difficult to make someone learn something if he does not want to learn it. For example, an activities therapist might set up several role-playing sessions in which patients place and answer a variety of different kinds of telephone calls. Whether a given patient, even with added practice, actually learns how to use a telephone is up to him. It appears that learning can be forced only when the teacher has total, life-and-death control over the learner's environment. Naturally, this is neither the usual nor the desired situation in activities therapy. The patient-learner is free to learn or not to learn. This is one of his basic privileges. A therapist can only help a patient *want* to learn.

A beginning therapist often raises the question of why the patient should be encouraged to change if he shows no interest in altering his behavior. The best answer is that most patients cannot participate fully in the life of the community. Unless they learn how to participate, they cannot freely decide whether they want to participate. For example, Matilda is not free to make the decision that she does not want to work when she has not acquired even rudimentary work habits. Without adequate work habits, Matilda has no real choice: She cannot work. The therapist is not taking away the patient's freedom; the therapist is allowing the patient to be more free.

In addition to knowing how to design learning experiences (to be discussed in the next section), a good teacher has two important attributes. First and foremost, a good teacher *likes* the learners with whom she is involved. A therapist must like her patients. If a therapist finds that she has negative feelings about a patient, she searches for the reason(s) for these feelings. Sometimes just finding the reason dissolves the negative feeling. At other times the therapist must work at developing liking for the patient. This is often done by getting to know the patient as well as possible. If all else fails, the therapist, after consultation with the patient, has another therapist take over responsibility for the patient. If this cannot be done, the therapist must be as open and honest as she is able with the patient about her feelings. It is silly to try to hide this sort of thing from a patient: He is bound to pick it up.

A good teacher always remains in the role of a teacher. The therapist never acts like a mother, a friend, or an older brother. This is particularly important for a therapist to remember. A patient sometimes begins to act as if the therapist were someone who is now, or was in the past, a significant person for the patient. The therapist may inadvertently take on the role the patient expects. For example, Jim's father had always made demands, but he would give in later and not require that Jim follow through on these demands. Through subtle cues, Jim indicated that he expected and wanted the therapist to act in the same way. If the therapist did what Jim wanted, she would be moving out of the role of a therapist and into the role of Jim's father. Treatment would essentially be discontinued. The therapist and Jim would simply become involved in a replay of Jim's family situation.

In psychoanalytic jargon, the patient shows *transference* if he acts as though the therapist is some person who was or is significant to him. The therapist who takes on the role desired by the patient shows *countertransference*. In psychoanalytically oriented therapy, transference is encouraged and used to explore past events. Activities therapy, however, does not utilize transference, because this type of therapy does not require exploration of past events. If it does occur, the therapist points out to the patient that his ideas about and expectations for the therapist are not appropriate to the situation. Other, more useful ways of relating to the therapist are suggested and encouraged. One way of keeping transference to a minimum is simply for the therapist to be herself. The therapist establishes and maintains her identity. This is done, for example, by letting the patient know early in the relationship that you are married to a man who teaches English in a high school, have two teen-age children, and live in such and such a neighborhood. Everyday events of the therapist's life outside the treatment facility are shared with patients. This personal presentation of the self differs from the psychoanalytically oriented therapist, who tries to encourage transference. This type of therapist tells the patient nothing about herself and attempts to maintain a neutral personality. This encourages transference because the patient, knowing little about the therapist, tends to develop ideas about her that are consistent with his past experiences with people who have been important to him.

The activities therapist acts similarly to the psychoanalytically oriented therapist in trying to avoid countertransference. This is accomplished by continual, conscious review of how one is relating to the patient. This may be done by asking such questions as: "Am I acting toward this patient any differently than I usually act with patients? Am I making different demands or concessions, or do I feel differently about this patient?" Identifying countertransference interactions with a patient is sometimes difficult. The therapist moves into a countertransference relationship rather slowly, taking the role expected by the patient unknowingly, almost as if the role were a natural one for the therapist to take. Because of the inadvertent aspect of forming countertransference relationships, it is often useful for the therapist to review her interactions with patients with fellow therapists or her supervisor or both. Another person, who is not working directly with a particular patient, is often able to see aspects of the patient-therapist relationship of which the therapist is unaware. Through such feedback, the therapist is able to make changes in her behavior toward or ideas about a patient.

Remaining in the role of a therapist does not mean that the therapist cannot "be herself." The therapist's own unique qualities and ways of relating to others are maintained as part of her role as a therapist. The therapist role of teacher, guide, and helper are integrated into other aspects of the therapist's personality. Being a therapist, admittedly, seems somewhat strange at first. One tends to feel like an actor playing a role. But the role soon becomes part of the self; it comes to be a natural and comfortable way of interacting.

What is a good learner? Probably someone who is motivated to learn. But motivation is an elusive quality. It seems to have more to do with the learning situation than with some predetermined orientation of the learner. In other words, with effort and studied consideration, a learning situation can usually be designed so as to catch the attention and interest of an individual. The next section describes some of the factors that contribute to the development of good learning situations.

PRINCIPLES OF THE TEACHING-LEARNING PROCESS

The principles outlined in the following pages are not rules, but rather ideas to be considered when the therapist is thinking about what she can do to help a patient learn to function in a more satisfying manner. One principle may be more important for the learning of a specific patient than another principle. For example, Jeff may learn more easily if he receives considerable feedback about how well he is doing, but Stacy may need the opportunity to set her own goals. Each person has his own way or style of learning. Part of being a therapist is to find out what will help each patient to learn. The following principles can be used as a guide.

1. *A good teacher begins where the learner is and moves at a rate that is comfortable for the learner.* This principle is probably self-evident, but it does need to be emphasized. One of the major mistakes therapists make with patients is to assume that they are able to do things they are really

not able to do. Treatment is often begun at a level far above where the patient is. For example, a patient who is not able to maintain any interest in what is going on around him is not going to be able to participate in an active game of volleyball. Rather, he may need a one-to-one situation in which the therapist makes a concentrated effort to maintain the patient's attention.

The kinds of ideas, skills, and values that a patient needs to acquire often take a long time to learn. The rate of learning may be very slow, and at times it may look as though no learning is taking place. Patients may go through periods in which there does not seem to be any change, and then suddenly begin to learn again. Some patients appear to need these "rest periods" to integrate or put together what they have already learned before they are able to go forward in the learning process. The difficulty is in trying to determine whether a patient is experiencing a "rest period," whether there is something in the treatment situation that is interfering with his learning, or whether he just cannot advance any further in that particular area. Sometimes the only thing a therapist can do is wait and see, make some changes in the learning situation, and wait some more.

However, it is not to be assumed that all patients learn slowly. Many patients advance very quickly in the development of desired abilities. If not prepared for such movement, the therapist may retard the growth of a patient. For example, Rita remained in a simple parallel-group treatment setting long after she had learned to function well in that type of group. Several weeks of valuable treatment time were wasted by not moving Rita into a more advanced type of group.

2. *A good teacher takes into consideration the learner's inherent capacities, age, sex, interests, assets and limitations, and cultural group membership.* One inherent capacity that must be taken into consideration is the intelligence of the patient. This does not mean the therapist needs to know the patient's IQ down to the last point. Rather, the therapist determines, in a general way, how bright the patient appears to be. If the patient seems to be below average intellectually, the therapist may find it necessary to use more simple words in talking with the patient and carefully select activities that are compatible with the patient's abilities. Another important inherent capacity is energy level. We are not discussing hyperactivity and hypoactivity here, but energy level in the normal range. There is wide variation in the amount of vigorous physical activity a person seems to need. Some people are tired after a game of shuffleboard, while others may

immediately want to play a second game of basketball. Similarly, some people can sit for long periods of time doing an intricate task or participating in lengthy emotional discussions, while others respond to such situations after a period of time by saying, "I have to get out of here and *do* something." Although such a response may be avoidance, it may also be that the person simply cannot tolerate being physically inactive for so long. Other factors included under the heading of "inherent capacities" are physical health, how well a person is able to see and hear, loss of sensation, degree of coordination, and the like. Difficulties in any of these areas are taken into consideration in planning a learning experience.

"That's for kids," or "a woman my age would never . . . !" might be heard in a treatment setting where the age of patients is not given sufficient attention. It is not always age *per se* that is important, but what activities people *think* are appropriate for various age groups. Some people feel that only children use finger paints, that middle-aged women do not roller skate, and that only old men play cribbage. Set ideas about relationships between age and activities are usually not dealt with in the treatment situation unless a patient has such narrow ideas of what activities are appropriate for his age group that he is unable to satisfy his needs. The therapist respects her patients' ideas about age and appropriate activities and seeks out activities her patients believe are suitable to their age. This is not to say, however, that the therapist cannot gently encourage patients to try some activities to which they originally responded to with, "That's kid stuff." Adolescents and young adults, as an age group, often have special activities they enjoy. As of the date of this writing, folk rock music and sewing fancy patches on blue jeans are big. For many, special activities of this age group serve as a source of identity and as a way of setting themselves apart from the older generation. Adolescents and young adults often learn more easily in a situation that makes use of activities that are currently popular in the youth subculture. It is helpful if the therapist keeps track of this rapidly changing scene.

There has been a rapid change in many cultural groups regarding what activities are appropriate for women and men. The women's liberation movement has altered many people's thinking about sex roles both in the family and the wider community. However, not everyone's ideas have changed. Some still believe strongly in the difference between "women's work" and "men's work." The whole issue of sex roles will probably remain a lively topic for discussion in treatment centers for some time to come. Given the current situation, the therapist should be extrasensitive to a patient's feelings about engaging in activities traditionally thought of as being "feminine" or "masculine." Ideally, one creates an atmosphere in which, for example, Rick, in attempting to learn how to organize a task, feels free to make either a shirt or a wooden shoe rack.

Difficulties arise in a learning process when a person is not interested in the activity being used to enhance learning. If Teresa does not like working with clay, this activity will probably not help her discover what ideas she has about herself. Some people are interested only in activities that have a useful end product. Others are interested in activities with creative aspects. Still others do not like activities that involve competition. And still others may want to engage only in activities that are "socially relevant." The more interested a person is in an activity, the more likely he is to learn what the activity was designed to teach him.

A person learns more easily if he is encouraged to do the things he does well in conjunction with learning something new. For example, Norm played the drums very well. This ability was used in helping him to deal with his ambivalent feelings about taking an authority role. Norm was encouraged and helped to take over the leadership of a newly organized quartet. As another example, Gill had never held a job. However, he did speak clearly and was able to use the telephone. These assets were used to get him into an on-the-job training program for telephone operators as a way of introducing him to the world of work.

A good teacher is concerned with the cultural background of the learner. One reason for this concern is that a therapist never tries to change a patient's values or ideas that are a traditional part of his cultural group. A person who is trying to learn how to function effectively in a community, which is usually made up of members of his cultural group, does not need someone to begin raising questions about the mutually shared values and ideas of his cultural group. Rather, he needs someone to help him learn how to live within the limits of these values and ideas. There are, however, a few occasions when an activities therapist is concerned with helping a patient change his culturally based values and ideas, such as when a patient has values and ideas so different from those of the broader community that they interfere with his need satisfaction or the rights of others, or when a patient sincerely wishes to become a member of another cultural group. These situations are, however, relatively rare.

In order for the therapist to know how to respect the orientation of a cultural group that is different from her own, the therapist must become familiar with the cultural group. Some areas for study include the following.

Importance of time: Ideas vary from "One must always be on time for everything," to "I have all the time in the world, so I'll get there when I get there."

Orientation in time: Some cultural groups are rooted in the past: Traditional ways of thinking and acting are the best. Other cultural groups are concerned only with the present: They feel the past is unimportant, the future is unknown, so it is best to enjoy and live in the present. Still other cultural groups are future-oriented. Saving money for a rainy day or old age, ultimately raising one's status in society, being recognized as having made a significant contribution to the community are examples of the beliefs of a future-oriented cultural group.

Political ideas: On what issues does a cultural group take a liberal view, and in what areas do they take a more conservative point of view?

Family: In some cultural groups the extended family (grandparents, aunts, cousins, etc.) is the most important unit. Basic loyalties and responsibilities are to the family. The nuclear family (father, mother, and children) is the significant unit for other cultural groups. Still other cultural groups do not see the family as being particularly central to one's personal life. Ideas about family also include who is supposed to have the last word. For some, the male members of the family make all important decisions about family matters. In other cultural groups, women exercise the ultimate power. Sometimes the decision is not that clear cut; in some areas women decide what is best, in other areas men have this prerogative.

Group versus the individual: In some cultures the group is the most important element. The group may be the family or an aggregate of peers. What the group decides is good; to be accepted one must go along with the group. In a cultural group with this orientation, competition between group members is usually not acceptable. Other cultural groups insist that the individual is all-important. They feel that each person should and must go out into the wider community and succeed or fail on his own merit.

Attitude toward other cultural groups: Attitudes toward other cultural groups vary from a feeling of kinship to indifference to hate. Stereotyping often plays a part in these attitudes: People who belong to some other cultural group are not seen as individuals with unique personalities but rather as persons who have characteristics shared by all members of the cultural group.

These are just a few of the cultural differences that exist in our society. There are many others. Developing understanding of another cultural group is not easy. One's own culturally based ideas and values come to be questioned. It is unsettling to learn that others have a world view that is very different from one's own world view. Accepting the legitimacy of the orientation of other cultural groups is difficult. It takes study, help from others, and a broadening of one's ideas about what values and ideas are "good" and "bad."

3. *The learner should be an active participant in the learning process.* This principle of the teaching-learning process is central to activities therapy. Verbal therapies involve discussions about problem areas and difficulties in doing. Activities therapy encourages patients to act in order to discover the nature of problem areas and to attempt behavioral change within the immediate situation. "Active participation" refers not only to learning through the experience of doing, but also to participation in planning the learning experience.

Role playing is a good example of learning through doing. Role playing involves two or more people acting out real-life situations. The purpose is either to understand these situations better or to practice some new type of behavior or both. As an example of the former, suppose Clare takes her own role as a wife while Sam plays the role of her husband as Clare has described him. They act out an incident that had occurred between Clare and her husband the evening before. In this replay of the interaction, Clare is able to experience again the emotions of the past evening and how she acted in response. After the immediacy of the role-playing period, Clare is helped to identify her emotions and discover in what ways she had influenced her husband's response toward her. With this new information Clare may be able to go home and deal with similar situations in a more appropriate manner. More typically, the learning experience continues as Clare is helped to identify more satisfactory ways of expressing her emotions or things she might do to alter the home situation so the strong emotions are not aroused in the first place. Clare may try out these ideas in additional role-playing incidents with Sam, both to decide if the agreed-upon behavior might be effective and to practice the new behavior. Alternatively, Clare might take the role of her husband. Taking an opposite role often helps a person to understand how his behavior affects others.

Other examples of the learner being an active participant in the learning process are Dedra going to the local "Y" to see if they have any activities she might enjoy, Philip taking charge of the bulletin board in order to develop a sense of responsibility, Gary making a link belt as a beginning step in developing task skills, Mary Jo playing checkers as a means of understanding why she is so competitive, and Sheila collating hospital center forms to develop work habits. Active participation means that a person is fully there in the learning situation. He is not being taught; he is learning.

4. *The consequence of an action is important.* What happens after a person has done something strongly influences whether or not he is likely to repeat the behavior. If the act led to need satisfaction, it is likely to be repeated. If the act led to need deprivation, it is not likely to be repeated. The term *reinforcer* is used to designate any event that increases the frequency of a particular act. A reinforcer is something that is ultimately need satisfying. Some common reinforcers are attention, approval, respect, a sense of mastery, a feeling of accomplishment, money, and food.

Behavior that is not reinforced tends to drop out of a person's usual pattern of behavior. For example, Marian may always have received attention and sympathy when she complained of vague aches and pains. If all the people in Marian's immediate environment stop giving her attention and sympathy when she complains, but instead give her approval for other things she does, Marian may stop talking about her aches and pains. The above is not only an example of eliminating a type of unwanted behavior, but it is also an example of differential reinforcement. *Differential reinforcement* is a process whereby a person is given reinforcement for one kind of behavior and not given reinforcement for another type of behavior.

One common way of learning is through the process of *shaping*. Shaping is a process whereby successive approximations of the desired behavior are reinforced. Successive approximation refers to increasingly more accurate attempts at doing something correctly. A toddler learning how to walk or feed himself is a good example of successive approximations. A therapist may use shaping to help a patient learn how to make his bed. At first the therapist gives approval or some other reinforcement for any attempt at making the bed. Later, approval is given only if the sheets and blankets cover the bed. Still later, the therapist gives approval only if the sheets and blankets are straight on the bed with no wrinkles. Finally, reinforcement is given only when the bed is completely and neatly made.

Many people feel that punishment or other need-depriving events should not be used in the teaching-learning process. One reason for this belief is that punished behavior does not seem to drop out of a person's usual pattern of behavior: He only gives up the behavior in these circumstances where he is likely to be caught. Another reason is that fear of punishment or need deprivation can be so severe that a person may stop trying to learn. For example, a therapist who makes critical remarks to patients in a discussion group may find that the patients eventually refuse to discuss anything at all. When a person knows that he is going to be punished if he makes a mistake or does not always live up to the demands of others, he is likely to try to avoid the situation entirely.

In the initial stages of learning, the individual often needs a considerable amount of reinforcement. Less reinforcement is usually needed later on in the process. Ideally, movement from frequent to infrequent reinforcement is gradual. Abrupt changes in the amount of reinforcement may interfere with the learning process.

One of the major concerns of the therapist is finding what will work as a reinforcer for a patient. Not all patients respond to attention and approval. This is particularly true for patients who have been hospitalized for a long period of time or patients who are extremely withdrawn. Candy, gum, or cigarettes sometimes serve as reinforcers for patients who presently seem to be experiencing only very primitive needs. As treatment progresses, the therapist slowly substitutes less concrete reinforcers such as attention and approval. Reinforcement used in the teaching process is ultimately designed to be similar to the kind of reinforcement that is available in everyday life.

Use of reinforcement is responsible for the development of a "token economy" in some treatment centers. Token economy is the name given to a way of structuring the treatment setting. Patients are given tokens for appropriate behavior, attending meetings, working on the ward, getting to the center on time, and so forth. These tokens can then be exchanged for food, permission to attend recreational events, passes, and the like. Some people object to this type of treatment because they feel that token reinforcement is too artificial. They say that this kind of reinforcement is too different from the kind of reinforcement available in the wider community. This is true in some respects. But token economy treatment centers that are effective also provide a considerable amount of nonconcrete reinforcement (i.e., attention, affection, compliments, etc.). Effective centers also plan the giving of tokens according to the learning needs of each individual patient.

Learning in many areas is enhanced by feedback. *Feedback* is the information one receives about the way one's own behavior affects other people or things. It is a useful device in the teaching-learning process. Many times a person does not know how his behavior affects others. He needs information about what other people think and feel about his behavior. The actions and responses of others frequently provide nonverbal clues about the effect of behavior. But reading these clues is often difficult. Thus it is useful to have another person give feedback verbally. People also need information about how they are doing in the learning situation. "Am I doing all right?" "Is this right or wrong?" These are common questions of any learner. Answering these questions (even if they are not asked directly) provides the learner with valuable information.

5. *Opportunity for trial and error and imitation enhances learning. Trial and error* is responding to a new situation with a variety of goal-directed acts. The motivated learner keeps trying until he finds something that works. Trial-and-error responses may be overt and visible to an observer, or they may be covert, in that the person thinks about various courses of action. People are more likely to engage in trial-and-error learning if they are in a setting in which mistakes and false starts are seen as a normal part of the learning process. There should also be plenty of time to work things out. Trial and error involves figuring things out for oneself rather than being told. Many people prefer this way of learning.

Imitation is responding to a new situation by copying the actions of another person more or less exactly. The crucial factor in imitation is to have good models for imitation. Faulty models lead to faulty learning. In a treatment center, for example, a staff who is not able to express emotions adequately or resolve conflicts among themselves is going to have a hard time helping patients develop these skills. Models for imitation are usually selected by an individual for two reasons: He likes and respects the other person and wants to be more like him, or he sees that the other person's behavior is effective in getting something that he himself wants.

6. *Frequent repetition or practice facilitates learning.* Hardly anyone develops a complex skill by practicing the skill only a few times. The behavior implicit in the skill has to be repeated many times in order for it really to become part of a person. It takes considerable repetition before a skill is so well learned that one can do it automatically without having to think about it. The skills that patients hope to learn are very complex.

Unfortunately, they are not always given enough time to practice these skills. Patients are sometimes discharged before they have had enough time to integrate new learning. Dan, for example, finally learned to function fairly well in his protective and supportive ward group. However, when he returned to the community he again began to have difficulties participating in groups. It may well be that he had not had sufficient time to make group-interaction skill a part of his usual behavior.

The importance of practice points to the desirability of there being many treatment activities available for patients. Patients cannot learn very much if they only receive help with their learning one or two hours a day. This is not to say that patients do not need time for relaxation; they do. But in many treatment centers patients spend far too much time in meaningless activities or doing nothing.

7. *Learning goals set by the learner are more likely to be attained than goals set by someone else.* As will be emphasized again in Chapter 6, the activities therapist and the patient together set the goals for treatment. This is true for the long-term goals of the whole treatment process as well as for short-term goals set along the way. Goal setting by the patient tends to give him an additional sense of responsibility and participation in the treatment process.

Occasionally problems arise when a patient sets unrealistic goals. They may be too high, as in the case of Leo, who was 35 years old and had never held a job for more than three months at a time but wanted to be able to own his own business. Or they may be too low: Cynthia, for example, was 17 years old and had done well in school up until a month before she requested help at the day treatment center. She stated her goal as, "I want to be able to spend my time at home reading and watching TV without hearing the voices in my head." The therapist must spend considerable time helping patients who set unrealistic goals. For patients who set goals that are too high, the therapist often accepts that goal for the present. She then helps the patient focus on an immediate goal that is more reasonable for him to work toward at the present time. For the patient who sets goals too low, the therapist describes the things the patient has been able to do in the past and the things he is able to do even now. He is strongly encouraged to select, at least temporarily, a goal that is more in keeping with his potential.

Some patients are functioning at such a primitive level that they cannot set goals for themselves. In this case the therapist must take responsibility for setting goals. The therapist tells the patient what the goals are even if it appears that he really does not understand. Later, when the patient is able, the therapist talks with him about what goals he has for his treatment. Patients sometimes need help in formulating goals. They may have a general idea about what they would like to do in the future, or the kind of person they would like to be. However, the patient may not be able to identify the specific things he is going to have to learn how to do in order to function independently. The therapist *helps* the patient express his goals. She does not force her ideas upon him.

8. *Practice in different situations encourages generalization and discrimination.* Generalization is here defined as the ability to apply what was learned in one situation to another appropriate situation. Discrimination is the ability to determine what is appropriate behavior for one situation as opposed to another situation. Together, generalization and discrimination are the ability to match behavior to the situation. The therapist can help a patient to function in the treatment setting, but it is far more important that he be able to function in the community. Thus she is interested in the patient transferring what has been learned in the treatment center to his daily life in the community. As the principle indicates, practice in different situations helps a person learn what behavior to use in a variety of different circumstances. This can be done in the treatment center, for example, by encouraging a patient to apply newly learned task skills to all tasks he is asked or required to perform. Discrimination might be enhanced by helping a patient realize what tasks require considerable attention to detail and what other tasks demand much less concern for details.

By far the best way of ensuring transfer of learning to the wider community is for the patient to live in the community while participating in the treatment process. If a patient is able to go home in the evening or at least on weekends, or if he works during the day and spends his evenings and nights at the treatment center, he has an opportunity to try out new behavior. Difficulties in using newly learned skills or not knowing whether one response is better than another can be talked about while the situation is still fresh in the patient's mind. Patients who remain in the treatment center for long periods of time without any contact with the world outside have no way of knowing if they have really gained new knowledge, skills, and values. And neither does the therapist. Treatment is taking place in a vacuum. Many patients learn how to function in a treatment center, but remain totally inept at functioning in the real world. Patients must have an opportunity to try new ways of acting in an unsheltered situation. If they do not, the sheltered situations may be a hindrance to rather than a help in furthering their growth.

9. *The learner should understand what is to be learned and the reasons for learning.* One good way of finding out if this teaching-learning principle is being used is to talk with patients after an activities therapy session. If the majority of patients are unable to say why they were participating in the session or what they expected to gain from participation, it is fairly safe to guess that the full potential of the activities therapy session is not being utilized. Minimal learning takes place if a person does not know what he is supposed to learn or why he is being encouraged to learn something new. There seems to be a belief among some mental health workers that the less a patient knows about what he is expected to learn the better. These workers think that if a patient knows what he has to learn to be a better functioning person, he will resist learning. They feel that the therapist must somehow "sneak up from behind" in order for learning to take place.

Ideally, the therapist demonstrates or at least describes in detail what she expects the patient to learn. Further, the therapist explains how learning of this particular skill, information, or value will lead to the previously set goals. For example, one way of helping people learn how to participate in a nurturing relationship is to encourage them to care for plants or an animal of some kind. If the patient does not understand how the nurturing demands of plants and animals relates to his desired goal of getting involved in the care of his infant son, he will probably feel that the activity is meaningless. Some of the important points—"What do I get in return?" "Who is going to take care of these nonhuman things while I am away for the weekend?" and "They certainly are demanding and take up a lot of my time"—will never be brought into focus because the patient does not understand the purpose of the activity. Opportunities for exploration of ideas and skill learning are lost. The therapist who asks herself, "What would it be like if I were placed in a situation where I was supposed to learn something but did not know what nor why" is well on the way to understanding this principle of learning.

10. *Planned movement from simplified wholes to more complex wholes enhances learning.* This principle is a modification of the idea that learning is enhanced if one moves from the simple to the complex. The idea of

wholes is emphasized here to remind the reader that learning should not move from arbitrary, meaningless *parts* to meaningful wholes. For example, if a patient has had no experience in using a public transit bus, it is better to organize the learning experience so that learning how to ride a bus is taught within the context of getting ready to go somewhere, getting there, and engaging in some pleasurable activity at the end of the journey. Just taking a bus ride for the sake of learning how to use public transportation is breaking an activity into meaningless parts.

In thinking about designing a learning experience, the therapist analyzes what is to be learned. This should be done in terms of graduated levels of what is to be learned rather than in terms of the isolated skills and knowledge to be acquired. Consider, for example, the task of teaching a patient to be self-sufficient in taking care of his need to eat every day. The knowledge and skills needed are (1) being able to plan what to buy given one's budget and basic nutritional needs, (2) getting to the grocery store, (3) finding the desired items, (4) paying for the items and getting the right change back, (5) getting home, (6) storing the food properly, and (7) fixing a meal. The next question to be asked is, "What is the simplest level at which all of these things can be taught?" Teaching in isolation each of the tasks outlined above fragments learning; the meaningful wholes are lost. Ideally, beginning learning in this area would go something like this: The patient and therapist talk about what the patient had for breakfast and the menu posted for the evening meal. On the basis of this information, the therapist helps the patient decide what to have for lunch. Information about nutrition is given in the context of planning. The therapist also tells the patient how much money they have to spend for lunch, so the decision of what to prepare is made within the confines of limited funds. The therapist tells the patient the location of the grocery store and how to get there. In the beginning stages of learning, the therapist will usually accompany the patient to the store. Likewise, at this level of learning, the patient buys only one item. He is asked to find one thing in the store. The patient and therapist together figure out how much change the patient ought to get back before the money and the item are presented to the cashier. Now the therapist encourages the patient to lead the way back to the treatment center. In the kitchen, the patient is asked to prepare only one of the more simple parts of the lunch, the therapist preparing the rest of the meal. Eating the meal should be a leisurely and enjoyable process. Again, in cleaning up, the patient is asked to do only one part. Within the context of cleaning up, the therapist helps the patient decide what would be the best way, for example, to store the cheese left over from lunch.

In the above example, the simplest aspects of each of the tasks that make up an activity of daily living were taught within the context of the total activity. Parts were not broken down and taught separately. All aspects were taught together to create a meaningful whole.

11. *Inventive solutions of problems should be encouraged as well as more usual or typical solutions.* There are few problems that have only one solution and few activities that must be performed in one specific way. Thus the learner should not be led to believe that there is only one right way of doing things. Rather, the learning situation promotes the idea that there are a number of ways of performing a task in a successful manner and that there are many modes of relating to people in a given situation. This is not to say that typical ways of dealing with things and events are never suggested: They are. Many of the patients the activities therapist treats are not able to engage in any sort of creative problem solving. Simply learning the usual ways of dealing with people and things is difficult for them. They need help in learning how to function, not in developing creative ways of functioning. For example, Rosemary, who is 50 years old, has been hospitalized for the last thirty years. In the hospital she is self-sufficient in activities of daily living and she holds a nonpaying job in the hospital cafeteria-style dining room, serving food from the steam table. Rosemary needs help in learning skills that are required for functioning in the community. She needs to learn about the community, she needs help in finding a place to live, she needs assistance in getting a job, she needs to learn to relate to her fellow workers. Learning all of this will be difficult enough. Rosemary does not need anyone to suggest that, in addition, she should do these things creatively.

On the other hand, there are patients who can profit from learning in an atmosphere that encourages divergent thinking. They can gain much from the opportunity to consider a variety of ways of accomplishing a particular task. Ruth, a 40-year-old woman with severe arthritis, for example, could not get her three teen-age children to give her the help she desperately needed in taking care of the household. Rather than spending money for outside help or continuing to yell at her children, Ruth assigned each child a task. The tasks were rotated each week. She never did the jobs she had assigned or said anything if they were not done.

The teen-agers began to complain to each other if there was no dinner ready or clean clothes to wear. They put pressure on each other to get the necessary tasks done.

Inventive solutions can be arrived at if such ideas as "It's always been done this way," or "Other people do it like this," or "You cannot change the system" are avoided. There should be a willingness to consider things from many directions. On the other hand, treatment centers, ideally, offer some structure, some sense of orderliness and consistency as well as general values about what is right and wrong. *Flexible structure* is perhaps a good way to describe a beneficial learning environment.

12. *There are individual differences in the ways anxiety affects learning.* Some people learn best when they are moderately fearful or anxious. Anxiety seems to motivate this type of person to get down to the business of learning. Other people can learn only if they are relatively free of anxiety. Even a moderate degree of fear seems to make them feel disorganized and unable to learn. For example, some people can only study for an exam the night before, while others prepare for the exam throughout the semester. Similar responses can be seen in a group of patients who have a specific date on which they must leave the treatment center. Some patients work steadily at eliminating their problem areas throughout the period of treatment. Other patients seem to idle away their time doing little to find solutions to their problems in functioning until the last few weeks of the treatment period.

The therapist attempts to identify the optimal level of anxiety for each patient and to regulate the learning situation accordingly. Richard, for example, could not tolerate the anxiety he experienced when he was supposed to get weighed each week. This was the usual practice at this treatment center for all patients, like Richard, who were on a reducing diet. The therapist arranged for Richard to be weighed only every six weeks. This diminished Richard's anxiety; he became much more comfortable about dieting, and it was easier for him to stay on his diet. On the other hand, Millicent could only continue to work on her difficulty of expressing feelings of liking and love if she was constantly reminded of her desire to be more open and affectionate with her husband and young daughter.

One difficulty in raising a person's anxiety level is that one is often tempted to threaten a decrease in need satisfaction or need deprivation. This comes very close to threatening punishment as a means of facilitating learning. As mentioned in the discussion about the importance to learning of the consequences of an action, it is probably best to avoid punishment in the teaching-learning process. The therapist must be inventive in trying to help a person who needs to be moderately anxious in order to learn. The patient and therapist often need to spend considerable time discovering ways of enhancing learning.

It is generally agreed that a high degree of anxiety interferes with learning. Only a very few people are able to learn when they are in a state of extreme anxiety or fear. About the only thing most people are able to do in a high-anxiety situation is to try to find a way out of the situation.

SUMMARY

This chapter has identified some of the factors within the teaching-learning situation that are believed to contribute to or enhance learning. One factor may be more or less significant for a particular patient. Some of the principles mentioned are probably more important for development of one facet of man than for development of another facet. The activities therapist designs or puts together learning experiences. She is concerned about how she will act, how she will present the learning problem to the patient, and about how the nonhuman environment should be structured in order to help the patient learn. Further, the therapist tells the patient how he can best make use of each learning situation. But it is the patient who must do the learning. It is he who brings about change in himself.

SUGGESTED READING

Bruner, James. *Toward a Theory of Instruction.* Cambridge, Mass.: Harvard University Press, 1966.

Clayton, Thomas. *Teaching and Learning.* Englewood Cliffs, N.J.: Prentice-Hall, 1965.

Hilgard, E., and Bower, G. *Theories of Learning.* New York: Appleton-Century-Crofts, 1966.

Hill, Winfred. *Learning: A Survey of Psychological Interpretations.* Scranton, Pa.: Chandler Publishing Company, 1963.

Jeffers, Camille. *Living Poor.* Ann Arbor, Mich.: Ann Arbor Publishers, 1967.

Komisar, P., and Macmillan, C. *Psychological Concepts in Education.* Chicago: Rand McNally & Co., 1967.

Leebow, Elliot. *Tally's Corner.* Boston: Little, Brown and Company, 1967.

CHAPTER 4

GROUP DYNAMICS AND PROCESS

As far as we know, man has always been a social being, living with others in a group. As previously mentioned, one of the skills basic to adequate functioning is the ability to get along in a group. Rejection from community groups (the family, work group, social group) interferes with need satisfaction. Being rejected from community groups and being unable to find other, substitute groups is often one of the major reasons a person seeks help at a treatment center.

The activities therapist needs to know what factors contribute to the maintenance of a productive group for two reasons: First, in order to help others learn how to function in groups, the therapist must have some idea of the information, skills, and values needed for good group participation. Second, the therapist uses groups for the development of many facets of the private and public self. The group provides the background for learning in these areas. Therefore, the therapist must know enough about groups to form a group that will contribute to learning. She must be able to look at an on-going group and decide if events occurring in the group are interfering with learning.

DEFINITION OF A GROUP

A group is an aggregate of people who share a common purpose which can be attained only by group members interacting and working together. Groups come into being because it is difficult or impossible for an individual to accomplish something alone. Groups form because people realize that they require other people to help them satisfy their needs.

Groups vary in size from a few persons to millions; a family may be made up of three or four people, while the Roman Catholic Church is a group of several million people. We are interested here only in small groups, that is, small in the sense that everyone in the group knows everyone else and that the group, as a whole, is able to sit together in a discussion. The activities therapist usually works with groups of from five to twelve people. She may, however, be involved in meetings where there are forty to fifty people. Fifty people is probably the maximum number for any group that could be called "small." It is very hard for a group of more than fifty people to sit together and discuss something, since some people are bound to become audience rather than participants in the group. There are certain dynamics and processes that have been identified for large groups, but these will not be discussed here.

Dynamics and process is commonly used to refer to various facets of small groups that are in a continuous state of change. Small groups are difficult to study and discuss as whole units. Groups are broken down into parts so that they may be examined more carefully. The facets of a group are interdependent, however, and all facets must be taken into consideration in looking at any particular group. It was once thought that most small groups are fairly static, that they change very little in the course of their life. We now know this is not true. Groups are usually active, ever-changing units. This chapter is devoted to a discussion of some of the dynamics and processes or facets of small groups.

GROUP MEMBERSHIP ROLES

Group membership roles refer to what people do in groups—to how people act. Several common group membership roles that seem to contribute to the well-being of a group have been identified. They are divided into two categories, *task roles* and *social-emotional roles.*[1]

Task roles are the roles that are usually needed for a group to select, plan, and carry out a group task. These roles are as follows:

1. The initiator-contributor, who suggests new ideas.
2. The information seeker, who asks for clarification of facts.
3. The opinion seeker, who asks for clarification of opinions or values.

---

[1] Talcott Parsons and R. Bales, *Family, Socialization and the Interaction Process,* New York: The Free Press of Glencoe, 1955.

What roles do I take in groups

4. The information giver, who offers facts.
5. The opinion giver, who states his beliefs or values.
6. The elaborator, who spells out suggestions.
7. The coordinator, who clarifies relationships.
8. The orienter, who defines the position of the group with respect to its goals.
9. The evaluator-critic, who compares the accomplishments of the group to some standard.
10. The energizer, who prods the group to action.
11. The procedural technician, who expedites group movement by performing routine tasks.

The second category, social-emotional roles, is concerned with the function of the group as a group and satisfaction of members' needs. These roles are as follows:

1. The encourager, who praises, agrees with, and accepts the contributions of others.
2. The harmonizer, who mediates differences between group members.
3. The compromiser, who changes his own behavior so as to maintain group harmony.
4. The gatekeeper, who facilitates and regulates communication.
5. The standard setter, who expresses standards for the group to achieve.
6. The group observer, who notes, interprets, and presents information about group process.
7. The follower, who goes along with the movement of the group.

The above roles are not the only roles a person may play in a group. Other roles, essentially the opposites of those above, interfere with the functioning of a group. For example, a person who gives no suggestions or stirs up conflict between group members gets in the way of the group doing what it wants to do. A person who takes roles that are detrimental to the group may simply not know how to contribute to a group. Or the individual may have a goal that is not compatible with the purpose of the group. For example, a person who wants to be the center of attention is not going to do well in a group that is meeting to review ward rules.

Ideally, an individual is able to take a variety of group membership roles. He moves from one role to another as the group situation demands. Thus, for example, he may start out, during a specific group meeting, as one of the persons acting as information givers. Later, he may feel that the group has enough information; they need to make a decision. Seeing that no one else is calling for the group to take action, he moves into the role of the energizer. Still later, he may find himself acting as harmonizer. A person who takes only one group membership role regardless of the situation probably does not know very much about group participation. Aside from being a bore, he usually makes little contribution to a group. A person who always acts as the evaluator-critic is a familiar example. Role flexibility is the desired quality.

What roles need to be taken in a group at a particular time will depend on the purpose of the group or where the group is in accomplishing a task or both. A group devoted to discovering the effect of one's behavior on others, for example, has less need for people to take the role of standard setter than it does for members to take the role of gatekeeper to facilitate and regulate communication. Standard setting, however, becomes increasingly important in a group devoted to the development of task skills. Similarly, for example, if a group is trying to decide on an activity, it needs people in the role of initiator-contributor to suggest new ideas and information giver to offer facts. Much later, when the specific activity is completed, the group needs orienters to define the position of the group with respect to its goals and evaluator-critics to compare the accomplishments of the group to some standard. As the examples indicate, the roles that need to be taken depend on the situation.

The reader may be more familiar with thinking about group roles in terms of leader and follower. Describing roles as membership roles places less of a division between leader and follower and more clearly identifies the roles needed for a group to move toward its desired goals. When a person is clearly taking the role of leader, he is generally taking the majority of the roles outlined above. There is less distinction between leader and follower when there is wide distribution of membership roles among group participants.

There are various ways of helping people learn how to take on group membership roles:

1. The designated group leader does not take all of the roles needed for a group to function in a given situation. He allows

the group to flounder a bit. This allows group members to experiment with roles; it increases the opportunity for trial-and-error learning.

2. The activities therapist and group members talk about the various membership roles and the way a person may act to fulfill these roles. Examples are given from past experiences in groups of people who took these various roles. There is also discussion of when one role is needed more than another.

3. At times, it is beneficial for a group to stop what it is doing and look at what roles have been taken in, say, the last half hour or forty-five minutes. This clarifies how a role is played, because the role was just taken. The situation or the needs of the group can also be examined. This helps the group participants determine if the taking of additional or different roles would be useful to the group at this time.

4. Role playing of group membership roles allows patients to experiment with roles without the pressure and demands of a real group situation. There is time to think about the role and try various approaches. Feedback from observers is also available.

5. It is sometimes useful for a person to watch a group as an outside observer. The group may be one in which the observer is usually an active participant, or it may be a group to which he has never belonged. This allows the individudal to see roles and the behavior necessary to fulfill a role from a less personally involved position. Participants in the observed group may serve as models for the observer when he once again takes an active part in a group.

6. A group member may be given special attention or praise when he takes on a role he has never before played in the group, or when he plays a role particularly well, or when he rescues a group from a dilemma by taking a role needed for the group to continue toward its goal. This increases the possibility that the person will take this role again.

In designing a learning situation, the activities therapist tries to determine what membership roles are likely to be needed in a group. She tries to decide what roles the patients will be able to take, and therefore what roles she should be prepared to play herself. From this point, the therapist remains flexible, moving in and out of roles as needed. As a general rule, the therapist takes as few membership roles as possible without letting the group wander aimlessly for any extended period of time.

DECISION MAKING

Decision making is the process of arriving at an agreed-upon solution to a problem. It involves deciding what course of action should or ought to be taken. Group decision making differs from individual decision making in that a number of people must come to an agreement about the decision. In individual decision making, the person decides what to do himself. He may have to worry about what others may think of his decison, but he makes it alone.

Group decision making has several phases. A group may go straight through each phase to the solution or it may move back and forth between phases. The first phase is identification of the problem. Sometimes this is the hardest part of the decision making. Group members may feel that something needs to be done or they may have a vague feeling that something is wrong, and yet remain stumped for days about what the problem is. For example, a patient government group became aware of the fact that, rather suddenly, many of the agreed-upon rules of conduct in the treatment center were not being followed. It took them considerable time to realize that the reason for the rule breaking was arbitrary enforcement of the rules. Sometimes a patient or staff member was penalized for disregarding a standard of conduct and sometimes he was not penalized. Proper identification of the problem is often a big step toward finding a solution to the problem.

The next step is getting information about possible solutions. How have other people solved the problem? What are the consequences of solving the problem one way as opposed to another way? This is an area in which divergent thinking may be encouraged. A traditional or usual solution can be set aside, at least for a time, while group members "brain storm" or offer any solution that comes to mind. Usually, the more information a group has, the more likely they are to arrive at a reasonable decision.

The third step is reaching a conclusion, that is, deciding what course of action to take. There are several ways of arriving at a conclusion. One way is by *unanimous decision,* full agreement by all group members regarding the best possible solution. In a unanimous decision, everyone agrees; no one is unhappy about the conclusion and there are no dissenters. This is a difficult type of conclusion to reach, especially if group members do not collectively share many values and ideas. Another kind of conclusion is *consensus,* in which the minority agrees to go along with the majority while maintaining the right to have the decision reevaluated at a later date. The minority says, "All right, we will do what most of the group wants to do, but if we still do not like the idea next week, we will call for further discussion regarding the decision." One of the problems with consensus is that the minority may not try very hard to implement the decision. They may use stalling tactics or attempt to sabotage what the group is trying to do. Under *majority rule,* another way of making a group decision, most of the group agree to one solution. The minority is expected to go along, and they do not have the right to demand reevaluation of the decision at a later time. This is probably the most common way of reaching a decision in our culture. It is considered part of the democratic way of life, but it often seems to be a cold, unfeeling process: Someone is always the loser. Groups that rely entirely on majority rule may find that members who always find themselves in the minority position drop out of the group. These persons may form their own group, in which their shared ideas have a chance of being accepted and acted upon. Total reliance on majority rule, however, may also affect patients in a somewhat different way. Patients often do not have the ability to form their own group. Those who are frequently in the minority may leave the group, and, because of the lack of group-interaction skills, remain isolated from the life of the treatment community. The one other way of reaching a decision is *compromise.* Compromise is the combining of two different solutions. The ultimate course of action is something quite different from either proposed solution. In compromise, if one faction of a group wants to go to the movie and the other faction wants to go swimming, they may ultimately end by going to a baseball game. In compromise, someone has to think of a third alternative that everyone finds agreeable.

Because there are so many different ways of arriving at a decision, it is usually necessary for group members to decide what kinds of decision making will be used in the group. When this is not clearly stated, a group may not know, in fact, if they have really reached a decision.

The final stage in decision making is implementation, that is, carrying out the solution. After a solution to the problem has been reached, group members work together to resolve the problem. For example, if a group decides to paint the hallway blue, someone has to do the actual painting. One of the best ways of determining whether a group has made a decision that took into consideration the needs and feelings of most of the group members is to look at its implementation. If a group does not carry out the agreed-upon decision, there was probably something wrong with the decision or the process by which it was reached. Unfortunately, there are many groups that decide to do something that never gets done. There is often more talk than action.

There are several factors that can interfere with decision making. One factor is fear of the consequences of making a particular decision or any decision. Group members may be afraid that other people, whom they see as powerful or important, will not like their decision. For example, in a community meeting at which the head nurse was absent, it was decided that roommates should determine how neat they wanted to keep their room. If they did not want to make their beds, hang up their clothes, keep things in drawers, and so forth, all they had to do was keep their door closed. Group members never acted upon this decision because the head nurse, who could be difficult when crossed, believed that order and neatness were all-important. Another consequence group members may fear is added responsibility. They do not want to do the work that a decision entails, or they believe that ultimately they will fail. An example of how fear of added responsibility may affect a group is a patient recreation committee that wanted to raise money to buy a movie camera. Every fund-raising project suggested was finally rejected because the group saw each project as overwhelming—too big or complex for the group to handle. Fear of change is another consequence that may interfere with decision making. A group may never find a solution to a problem because it is really comfortable with things as they are. What is familiar, even though somewhat disturbing, is seen as better than moving into unknown territory.

Talking about the possible consequences of a decision may help a group arrive at and carry out a decision. The things that might actually happen, as well as fantasies that individual group members may have, are discussed. Members are encouraged to express their fears openly. Shared fear tends to be less inhibiting to action than fear kept to oneself. The activities therapist gives extra support and encouragement to members who express anxiety.

The second factor that may interfere with decision making is conflicting loyalties. A person may be a member of two groups, each group having different ideas about how a problem should be solved. Kevin, for example, as a member of the safety committee, knew that his group was going to have to make some decision about community members bringing objects that might be used as dangerous weapons into the treatment center. Fights did occasionally break out. People were less likely to get badly hurt if there were no weapons available. However, Kevin also belonged to an informal subgroup of patients who carried switchblade knives. Because he was fairly sure the safety committee was going to decide that likely weapons must be left with the receptionist, Kevin tried to delay the decision by bringing up all sorts of irrelevant issues.

When some group members seem to have conflicting loyalties, the therapist can help by encouraging group members to talk about the two solutions. In this way the conflict is brought into the open. The individual can get help from other people as to how he might solve the conflict. It may be found, after examining the situation, that the differences are not really basic. Minor adjustments may solve the conflict. If conflicting loyalties cannot be resolved, the individual receives help both in deciding which group is more important to him and in leaving the less important group.

Decision making is sometimes hampered by interpersonal difficulties. One person may reject every proposal or idea another person presents because he does not like the other person. He does not weigh the merit of the suggestions offered; he will not accept them because they were made by someone whom he finds offensive. When there are interpersonal difficulties in a group, the group may divide into two factions. Each faction remains loyal to one of the two people who cannot seem to get along together. In this case the group often dissolves into petty bickering and discussion of irrelevant issues. No one is attending to the business of the group.

About the only way that interpersonal difficulties can be resolved is to bring them into the open. This is hard both for the two people in conflict and for the other group members. The individuals involved must be helped to talk out their differences and express their feelings about each other. Honesty is encouraged. Somehow the two individuals must learn to live with each other, at least within the group situation, or one person will have to leave the group. Hopefully, the therapist is able to avoid this eventuality. Unresolved personal antipathy festers like a hidden abscess. It is almost sure to disrupt the group at some point.

Decision making is a deliberate process. It should be given sufficient time and attention in any group. Quick decisions are often hard to live with in the future. Ideally, a group is never forced to make a decision before it is ready. Finally, it is important that a group make decisions based on the facts of the situation rather than purely on opinions or hearsay.

COMMUNICATION

Communication is the process of giving and receiving information by means of gestures, words, and tone of voice. (Written communication is not usually used in small groups, so it will not be discussed here.) Obviously, it is necessary for group members to talk freely with each other if a group is to remain a viable unit. Communication is used to clarify group goals, to identify problems in need of solution, and to resolve conflicting opinions or values. Communication is *clear* if there is general agreement among group members as to what everyone is saying. Communication is said to be *reciprocal* if it is a two-way as opposed to a one-way process. It is better for people to talk together rather than "talking to" or being "talked at."

One problem that may arise in communication is for a person to say one thing in words while at the same time saying something else by his gestures and tone of voice. Examples of such mixed communication are Irene saying she likes Matthew all right while moving away from him on the couch and giving him disgusted looks; Burt saying he is going to look for an apartment tomorrow in a flat, uncommitted tone of voice, and Jean saying "I didn't do it" while looking undeniably guilty. When a person is sending mixed messages, it is often useful to stop the conversation to find out which message he really intended sending. Many times people do not know they are sending conflicting messages: They are often unaware of what they are saying by gesture or tone of voice or both. This nonverbal message is usually the more accurate of the two.

The flow of communication is important in all small groups, but particularly in therapy groups. One common problem is that most of the communication is directed toward the therapist. The patients do not talk to each other, only to the therapist. If the therapist does not encourage conversation between patients, she is likely to end up participating in a series of one-to-one discussions. When this happens the group loses much of its potential for learning.

Lack of basic trust among group members inhibits communication. If a person does not know how others are going to react to what he has to say, or if he thinks he is going to get a negative response, he is probably not going to say very much. Lack of trust is common in a newly formed group, and it can often be seen in patients who have just recently arrived at the treatment center. There is a need to "feel out" the situation, to find out what people are like. Participating with others in an activity that allows for informal conversation tends to increase trust.

Group members who think of themselves as inadequate, inept, and fragile tend to have difficulty communicating. They often do not speak because they are afraid of revealing themselves. They do not want others to see what they are like. At the same time, other group members often avoid talking to patients who appear to have a poor self concept. They fear they may say something that will hurt the patient, and they have the idea that such a patient may "fall apart." A person who talks very little and is addressed only rarely cannot possibly feel that he is part of the group. The therapist can help the isolated patient by encouraging both the patient and the rest of the group to talk to each other.

Sometimes people communicate their ideas and values in an indirect manner. Thus, for example, one may hear such things as, "Some people feel . . ." when the person means "I feel," or "It's better to do it this way" when the person means "I think it is better to do it this way." A person who communicates indirectly is not taking complete responsibility for his own feelings, ideas, or values. He appears to be more comfortable in attributing these facets of himself to some vague "other." The therapist may help a patient to avoid indirect communication by reminding him to use "I" when he is speaking. Or she may, after a patient has made such an indirect statement, say, "Yes, but how do you personally feel about it?" A group that allows members to communicate in an indirect manner almost never gets beyond the level of being a social group; the private self is rarely touched.

Communication is the way in which a person makes contact with his fellow man. It is one of the principal means of gaining information about the world and giving information about oneself. The quality of communication, therefore, is a significant factor in any teaching-learning process.

GROUP GOALS

A group goal is the future state toward which a majority of the group's efforts are directed. A goal is what the group spends most of its time and energy trying to accomplish. The "true" goal, as it is defined in the last few lines, and the stated goal may be different. In other words, group members may say that their goal is one thing but spend most of their time doing something else. For example, members of an activities therapy group may say that the goal of their group is to learn more about their needs and emotions. However, they appear to spend most of their time making sandals for themselves; minimal time is spent in talking about feeling or in finding better ways to fulfill needs. The group's stated goal is not its real goal.

When an activities therapist uses groups for treatment, the goal of the group is to develop basic skills or facets of the private and public self. The goal is never to accomplish a particular task. One of the difficulties that activities therapists have is finding names for groups that reflect the goal of the group. They often end up with a title that has more to do with the activity to be used than with what is to be learned. One finds, for example, names such as "woodworking group," "cooking group," and "patient government group." It is only after discovering what goes on in a group that one is able to determine the goal. These activity-related names for treatment groups tend to confuse both patients and staff members who are not part of the activities therapy department. There is probably little that can be done to solve this problem until therapists become more inventive in thinking up names for activities therapy groups.

Goals both provide a point of orientation or focus for the group and set guidelines for group interaction. It is from knowing the goals of a group that the therapist is able to decide what activities might be appropriate, what kind of behavior she will encourage, and the kinds of things she might bring up for discussion. For example, if one of the goals of the group is to learn how to dress in a manner that is appropriate to the situation, the therapist may plan a series of activities that require different kinds of clothing. If the goal of the group is to develop work habits, the therapist will probably discourage lateness, talking about personal problems, and ingratiating behavior. If the goal of the group is to develop friendship relationships, the therapist might be prepared to discuss how to become acquainted with another person and how to ask someone to go to a movie.

Goals serve as standards by which a group may judge its activities, decisions, and progress. Knowing its goal of developing the capacity to make constructive use of free time, for example, the group may evaluate its effectiveness by finding out how many group members enjoyed their recreational activities during the past weekend. Group members, knowing the group goals, are able to decide if an activity will help them move closer to the goal. For example, a group with a goal of learning how to share responsibilities would probably decide that taking on the job of preparing lunch each Wednesday for the volunteers who come to the treatment center is a better activity for them than for each person in the group to make himself a pair of moccasins.

The stated goals of a group provide a reason for the group's existence for persons outside of the group and a means by which the outsider may judge the group. For example, a clay sculpting group was designed to help patients who had difficulty identifying the ideas they had about themselves. To reach this goal, the group decided first to make clay models of themselves. A visitor to the art room, seeing the human figures that had been produced, might say the group had not learned very much about clay modeling. If the visitor has a mistaken idea about the goal of the group, his judgment regarding the worth of the group is likely to be faulty.

Group goals and the activities used to reach a goal must be compatible with goals and means accepted as legitimate by the wider community. If there is conflict, people in the wider community may put pressure on the group to change its goals or activities, or they may attempt to dissolve the group. An activities therapist may find that the group goal of improving facets of the public self is not acceptable to members of the staff who have a psychoanalytic orientation. Such staff members often feel that difficulties in activities of daily living, work, and recreation will be resolved automatically when a person becomes aware of unconscious conflict. Psychoanalytically oriented staff members may also object to the means for reaching goals. They often emphasize the importance of talking about past events, but the activities therapist is concerned only with the present. The activities therapist may also meet resistance from staff members who are concerned primarily with the use of psychoactive drugs. Staff members with this orientation sometimes feel that medication is the only important part of the treatment process. They may think that the purpose of activities is just to keep patients busy while they are being regulated on drugs.

The real goal of a group gives the group meaning and identifies its reason for being, both for the members of the group and for the wider community. The goals of a group provide limits for the group in terms of the kinds of interactions that are considered appropriate and useful. Finally, group goals serve as a standard by which group members can judge the effectiveness of their interactions.

GROUP COHESIVENESS

Group cohesiveness refers to the degree of closeness group members feel toward each other and the value they place on the group. In a group with a high degree of cohesiveness, group members have a feeling of togetherness, a sense of liking for and loyalty to each other. Group members believe their group is particularly good or special in some way. The group is seen as better than any other similar group to which it is compared. In a group with a minimal degree of cohesiveness, group members do not care very much about each other. They show minimal concern for each other's needs and desires. Group members do not feel that the group is a very important part of their life. They generally place a negative value on the group. One of the best ways to identify the degree of cohesiveness of a group is to find out how often members are absent from the group. For the individual, group cohesiveness can be identified in terms of his attraction to and acceptance by the group. A person is usually attracted to a group if he thinks he can gain something by participation. A person is usually accepted by the group if the other group members believe he has something to offer to the group.

A relatively high degree of cohesiveness contributes to group interaction. There is a sense of liking, trust, and a desire to work together. A highly cohesive group tends to try to accomplish its goals. When a group is important to a person, what other group members say and feel comes to be important also. The individual wants to do what the group thinks he ought to do so that he will continue to be accepted by the group. On the other hand, a person who is accepted by a group will be given attention. His ideas and feelings are recognized and accepted by the group. A cohesive group has a strong influence over its members. This influence can be used to enhance the learning of each group member. A highly cohesive group provides a sense of security which enables group members to discuss personal matters and try out new behavior.

It is possible for a group to be too highly cohesive. This occurs when group members are so attached to each other that they spend most of their time together. They have little interest in the wider community and rarely interact with people outside their group. They may even exclude others from activities that have nothing to do with meeting the goals of the group. Patients need to be part of one or more cohesive groups, but they also need to participate in the life of the treatment center and ultimately in the life of the community. Involvement in an overly cohesive group interferes with the opportunity to try out new ways of thinking, feeling, and acting with a variety of other people in different situations.

Because a relatively high degree of cohesiveness contributes to patient learning, the therapist tries to attain this degree of cohesiveness in treatment groups. One way this can be done is by frequent group meetings. People who spend a considerable amount of time together tend to form into a cohesive group. A group that meets at least two hours every day will probably be more cohesive than a group that meets only twice a week for an hour or so. Another factor that increases cohesiveness is for group members to see themselves as having many similarities. A group that sees itself as sharing many things in common tends to be more cohesive than a group that emphasizes the differences among members. The therapist helps group members to identify what they share in common with each other. In forming a group or in suggesting to a patient that he join a particular group, the therapist takes into consideration such factors as the group members' sex, age, interests, assets and limitations, cultural backgrounds, and the like. If at all possible, the therapist tries to make groups homogeneous at least in some respects. Activities therapy groups seem to work better if patients have more in common than their particular area of difficulty.

Two other factors seem to increase group cohesiveness. One of these factors is competition with other groups. Competition pulls group members together around the idea of winning or doing a better job. Competitiveness tends to define the group in relation to an "out-group." Mild competitiveness between groups in a treatment center, such as which group prepares the best lunches, may not be harmful. More serious competition, however, tends to focus attention on the task of an activity group, with the result that the purpose of the task gets lost. Emphasis is placed on doing the task well rather than on what is to be learned through doing the task. The other factor that enhances cohesiveness is an increase in the status of the group in the wider community. People like to be associated with a group that has high status. Unfortunately, however, wherever there are high-status groups, there must also be groups with lower status. Low-status groups are not particularly desirable in a treatment situation. Patients do not want to belong to a low-status group, and this is perfectly understandable. Rather than being concerned about increasing the status of a group, the whole activities therapy staff should work toward maintaining equal status for all groups. Any talk about one group being a better group than another group or that one group is "working" and another is not is carefully avoided.

An optimal level of group cohesiveness is sought by the activities therapist. Such a degree of cohesiveness contributes to the learning situation. The influence group members have on each other encourages learning. The patient who is learning slowly or is in a temporary crisis is given support; all the patients delight in the new learning of a group member.

GROUP NORMS

Norms are the value system of a group. Taken together, a group's norms are a statement of what that group believes is an appropriate way of thinking, feeling, and acting. When a person understands the norms of a group, he knows what is expected of him and he is able to predict what other group members will do. Group life is possible only because of norms.

Norms develop whenever a group of people interact over a period of time. The involved individuals decide what behavior is going to be accepted in this group and what behavior is not going to be accepted. This decision-making process may be at the verbal level: There may be much talk about what people can do in the situation, what they are not supposed to do, and what they ought to do. Or the decision-making process may be nonverbal: People decide what is and is not acceptable without actually talking about it. Often there is mixture of verbal and nonverbal decision making.

Groups develop norms because of man's need for safety. This need can be satisfied only by being in a situation in which one knows what he is supposed to do and what everyone else is likely to do. Without this knowledge, a person feels unsure of himself; he is afraid, and he feels threatened by the unknown. Groups cannot function if the members feel unsafe. Therefore, they lay down ground rules for how to act and establish a range of behavior that is considered acceptable by the group.

Group norms change over time. Change may be slow or rapid, but there always seems to be some change occurring. A change in norms may occur because the group has been confronted by behavior for which it has no norm. The behavior is new for the group, so they have never had any need to decide if it is good or bad. For example, Eliot, a homosexual, began wearing a dress and make-up to the day treatment center. No one had ever done that before, so the members and staff of the center had to decide whether this should be allowed. Alternatively, a new idea or additional knowledge may become available to the group and cause a change in norms. For example, Zelda, a patient in a long-term treatment center, came up with the idea that any patient who has been in treatment for three months may have a week's vacation from treatment if he desires. It had always been expected that a patient would stay in continual treatment until he was ready to leave. After discussion, this new idea was accepted. If staff members get vacation, why should not patients also have time off?

When a norm is ignored by most group members for a long period of time, it usually ceases to be a functional norm. For example, patients in one treatment center were traditionally expected to address staff members by their last names. Some patients began calling staff members by their first names. After a while, so many patients were doing so that the unwritten rule about addressing staff members was forgotten.

The norms a group develops may conflict with each other, with the goals of the group, or with the norms of the wider community. When there is conflict between two norms within a group, one norm is usually talked about and the other is tacitly agreed to by everyone but never discussed. An example of this is a group that firmly stated that it was all right to talk about *anything* in this group. However, no group member would dream of talking about his religious beliefs or personal money matters. When a group becomes aware of conflicting norms, they have to decide which norm they are going to live by. Thus, one group, for example, had to decide between "group members are responsible for the decisions they make" versus "group members who need medication and are not taking it on their own should receive medication by injection." The choice between norms is often difficult to make. One thing that a group does when they do not really want to make a choice between norms is to create another norm that prohibits recognition of the fact that the two norms are in conflict. They essentially agree to pretend that there is no conflict.

In most cases, when norms conflict with the goal of the group, either the norm or the goal of the group is changed. However, this cannot occur in a treatment group. If the goal is changed, the whole purpose of the group is lost. It is no longer a group devoted to bringing about a specific planned change in group members' ways of thinking, feeling, or acting. It becomes merely a social group or a work group. Therefore, the therapist has to help the group change the norm that is getting in the way of reaching the goals of the group. For example, in one group that had been designed to develop work habits, group members began to spend most of their time talking with each other, reading the newspaper, and going out to the canteen to bring back coffee and pastries. Everyone was having a good time, but there was little work being done. Group members were gaining very few work habits. After realizing what was happening, the therapist reviewed the goals of the group with the patients. They talked about the kinds of behavior that are acceptable in a work situation and what behavior is not acceptable. The therapist had to become more careful about enforcing group norms until the group members were able to take over this responsibility once again.

At times, the norms of a group may conflict with the norms of the wider community. For example, an activities therapy group may say that when a person experiences an urge to masturbate while he is in the group that it is perfectly all right and indeed a good idea to talk about these feelings. The norm of the treatment center may be that one does not talk about the urge to masturbate during everyday interactions on the ward. Another example is a treatment center where a person may express negative emotions in any way short of physically harming himself, another person, or property. The norms of the wider community usually have somewhat more strict limits as to what is an acceptable way of expressing negative emotions. The wider community may put pressure on a group to change a norm that the community does not accept. A group can either give in to this pressure and alter their norm or resist the pressure and continue to act in a way that they feel is beneficial for group members. If the latter course of action is taken, group members must learn to operate on a double normative standard. They must learn to act one way in the group and another way in the community.

When a person becomes a member of an on-going group, he must learn what the norms of the group are and how to act within limits of these norms. This learning process is called *socialization*. Socialization is learning about and learning to act in accordance with the norms of the group. People learn about norms by being told what they are and by observing what other group members say and do. A group usually allows a new member some period of time before expecting him to conform to all of the group's norms. A new member is not usually accepted as a full-fledged member until he has learned to act within the norms of the group. Once a person becomes a full-fledged member of the group, he is expected to enforce existing norms while he has at the same time the privilege of participating in the process of changing norms.

A group member who does not act in accordance with group norms is subject to "sanction" by other group members. *Sanction* is the term used to identify the process whereby a group tries to get one of its members to act within the limits of the group's norms. Sanctions may involve telling a person he is doing something that is not acceptable to the group, need deprivation, temporary dismissal from the group, a threat of punishment, or finally telling the person that he can no longer be a member of the group. If a person is strongly attracted to a group, he tends to give in to the pressure of sanctions and changes his behavior so that it is acceptable to the group. If he does not feel that the group is particularly important to him, he ignores the sanctions. He acts as he wants to act until he is finally rejected by the group.

Sometimes rejection by a group can be a valuable learning experience for a patient. But more often it is a negative experience, which leaves the patient feeling isolated and inadequate. The therapist usually tries to keep a patient from being totally rejected from a group. First, the therapist never suggests that a patient join a group that has norms the patient is unlikely to be able to accept. When a patient is having difficulty acting in accordance with the norms of the group, the therapist explains to the patient how the group norms can contribute to his learning and why the norms are reasonable and good. The therapist gives the patient extra support and encouragement. In addition, the therapist may ask the group to give the patient more time. She may explain to the group how and why the patient is having difficulty living up to the group's norms. She asks them to be patient and understanding.

There is no set formula of group norms that should be operant in an activities therapy group. What are good and bad norms are determined by what is to be learned from the group experience. For example, honest and free expression of emotions is a good norm for a group devoted to the development of facets of the private self. It is not a useful norm when the purpose of the group is to learn how to function in a work situation. Other norms are needed. The therapist must try to be continually aware of the norms of the group for which she is responsible. She must judge whether the norms are helping or hindering the learning of group members. If a norm is detrimental to learning, the therapist tries to change the norm.

SUMMARY

The activities therapist is much concerned about the dynamics and process of small groups. Small groups are used to help patients develop a greater understanding of who they are and what they are. They are used to help patients develop living skills needed for independent functioning in the community. By knowing about the intricacies of small groups and what patients need to learn, the therapist is better prepared to design learning experiences and to act as a leader-member of treatment groups.

SUGGESTED READING

Cartwright, D., and Zander, A. *Group Dynamics* (3rd ed.). New York: Harper & Row, 1968.

Hare, A., Borgatta, E., and Bales, R. *Small Groups: Studies in Interaction.* New York: Alfred A. Knopf, 1965.

Homans, George. *The Human Group.* New York: Harcourt, Brace and World, 1950.

Lifton, Walter. *Working with Groups.* New York: John Wiley & Sons, 1961.

Mills, Theodore. *The Sociology of Small Groups.* Englewood Cliffs, N.J.: Prentice-Hall, 1963.

Parsons, T., and Bales, R. *Family, Socialization and the Interaction Process.* New York: The Free Press of Glencoe, 1955.

CHAPTER 5

THE STRUCTURE OF
TREATMENT FACILITIES

This chapter is an introduction to psychiatric treatment centers. Psychiatric treatment is offered in a number of different kinds of centers, each with its own unique structure. These structures affect how the activities therapist works and how the activities therapy department fits into the overall structure of a treatment center.

EXAMPLES OF DIFFERENT KINDS OF TREATMENT CENTERS

Large State Hospitals

Large state hospitals are often a community in and of themselves. They are frequently found out in the country, away from metropolitan areas. State hospitals in many parts of the country are going through considerable change at the present time. An attempt is being made in some areas to do away with state hospitals entirely, locating treatment facilities directly in the community. This is being done because of the belief that patients will do better if they remain in their own community while receiving treatment. Continued contact with family and friends and familiar surroundings are believed to help the patient maintain his sense of identity and desire to become once again a full participant in the community. In other areas, it is felt that state hospitals will continue to exist but that there needs to be radical change in their structure and function.

Traditionally, state hospitals have a centralized structure. Staff members' first loyalty is to their own department (i.e., nursing, recreation, psychology, etc.). They are often moved from ward to ward as the need arises. When patients first come to the hospital, they go to an "admissions building." If a patient improves fairly rapidly, he is sent home. If a patient

65

does not improve, he is sent to another ward. To which specific ward he is sent usually depends on the level at which he is able to function. Patients are moved from ward to ward as their condition improves or worsens. Activities therapy does not usually take place on the ward; patients either go to the activities therapy building or to a room in their own building that has been set aside for activities therapy.

More recently, some state hospitals have developed a decentralized structure. A ward or a small number of wards are set aside for patients from a particular section of a city, a town, or a county. Patients are admitted directly to this ward and stay on the ward until they are discharged. The reason for this arrangement is that patients can be with people from their own community with whom they are likely to share common interests and experience. In addition, if a person needs to return to the hospital at some later date, he will be returning to familiar surroundings. Staff members are assigned to a specific ward, and it is expected that they will stay on that ward for an extended period of time. Their first loyalty is to the ward. Day-to-day work supervision is provided by the individual who is responsible for the ward. There continue to be departments of, for example, social work, but supervisors in the department structure serve more in an advisory or consulting capacity. They have little to do with the everyday work of the staff members. One or more activities therapists are usually assigned to each ward, or, if there is a shortage of staff members, one activities therapist may divide her time between two wards. Most activities therapy takes place on the ward. However, there may continue to be some centralized facilities, such as a sheltered workshop or a homemaking unit. Patients go to these special facilities if they need help, for example, in developing work habits or homemaking skills.

Decentralized state hospitals often either have or intend to develop satellite treatment centers in the community. A satellite treatment center is located in and serves the same community unit as the decentralized units of the state hospital. Staff members from the hospital work in the satellite centers. There is a close relationship between a ward and its satellite center. Staff members sometimes work part time on the ward and spend the rest of their time at the satellite center. Patients may receive out-patient treatment in the satellite center associated with their ward after they leave the hospital.

One of the major functions of the satellite center is to keep as many people as possible out of the state hospital. Several services are offered. The satellite center evaluates community members who come or are brought to the center to determine what kind of help they may need. People may be given on-the-spot help with a specific emotional problem. This type of assistance is sometimes called *crisis intervention*. Crisis intervention involves helping someone work out how to solve a particular difficulty. Advice, concrete assistance, and support are provided. Crisis intervention might be used, for example, to help Rosella, who came to the center distraught from sleepless nights and family conflict resulting from having to care for a rapidly deteriorating, senile father, or Ralph, who was upset and confused about what to do after his wife left him with the care of three small children. The satellite center sometimes refers people to other community agencies that are better prepared than the center to deal with a particular problem. For example, it might be suggested to Lucy that she take her mentally retarded daughter to a federally funded mental retardation center for further evaluation; or Gene might be told to go to a welfare agency office to see if he can get additional money to replace the overcoat he has lost. When a person is referred to another agency, he is often given help in making the first appointment and told to come back to the satellite center if the agency cannot help him.

Treatment is also available at a satellite center. This may involve participation in a full-time day treatment program or individual or group treatment once or twice a week for an hour or so. Only people who cannot possibly stay in the community while they are receiving treatment are sent to the state hospital. The principal criterion used in making this decision is whether or not the person is likely to do serious harm to himself or others. People who have returned from the state hospital may continue treatment for a time either in day treatment programs or in groups that meet periodically. There is also an opportunity to see a physician regarding changes in medication. Some satellite centers have a "maintenance" program. This is usually for people who have been hospitalized for a very long time and are able to make only a marginal adjustment to community living even with outside support. A maintenance program gives these people somewhere to go and something to do. Activities within the program are designed to maintain whatever abilities a person has, to keep him in contact with reality, and to help the individual meet his needs. Concrete assistance with daily problems in living is also available. Additional services other than those described may be available at some satellite centers; other centers may not offer all of these services.

Some state hospitals have developed "halfway houses." A halfway house is usually located in the community rather than on hospital grounds. It provides room and board for patients while they are adjusting to being in the community once again. A halfway house serves as a base of operation while the patient looks for work, a place to live, and compatible friends. There are usually staff members available at the halfway house to help the residents with their problems in adjusting to the community. There may or may not be an active treatment program.

At the present time, state hospitals that have decentralized many of their services are left with a limited number of short-term treatment wards for patients referred by satellite centers and a large number of, usually older, chronic patients. Many of these patients have physical illnesses as well as a severe deficit in living skills. The vast majority of this population will never return to the community. About the only humane thing that can be done is to help these people live out their lives in comfort. Programs for these patients are similar to the maintenance program described in the discussion of satellite centers.

Private, City, and County General Hospitals

The general hospital may have one ward devoted to the care of psychiatric patients or a whole wing of the building or some larger unit. There is often an emergency psychiatric service as well. The structure and programs vary considerably from one general hospital to another.

A general hospital with one or two psychiatric wards tends to have one of three methods of operation or some mixture of the three. First, the ward may only admit patients who have been referred by doctors allowed to admit patients to that hospital. The doctor continues to take responsibility for the patient, usually seeing him almost daily for individual verbal psychotherapy. There may or may not be an active treatment program for patients on the ward. One of the problems for a ward staff who want an active treatment program is that the ward program is often seen as secondary in this setting and inferior to individual psychotherapy. Patients either tend to be uninterested in a planned program of treatment on the ward or they see it only as a good way to pass the time. Length of hospitalization varies from a few days to two or three months.

The second common method of operation in a general hospital is to admit both patients referred by their private physicians and those who come to the emergency psychiatric service who are in need of hospitalization. All patients are evaluated and treated by ward staff members. Private physicians do not treat their patients while they are in the hospital but may, of course, resume treatment after the patient is discharged. Patients usually stay in the hospital for more than a few days, but they rarely stay for more than a few months.

The third method of operation is the use of psychiatric wards primarily for evaluation. Based on this evaluation, staff members may decide to send the patient to a state hospital, a state hospital satellite center, some other day treatment center, another community agency, or they may decide to give the patient psychoactive drugs until the right drug and dosage are found and then send him out into the community without further treatment. Treatment other than the use of psychoactive drugs may or may not be available on this type of ward. Often there is a program to keep patients active and busy during the time of their hospitalization, but this is not treatment. If there is a treatment program, it is usually concerned primarily with enhancing basic skills, work habits, and activities of daily living. Patients generally remain on the wards from two weeks to a couple of months. Patients who stay for more than a month often do so because there is some difficulty deciding where they should go or in getting a place to accept the patient.

General hospitals with larger psychiatric facilities most often use a combination of the three methods of operation described above. However, there does seem to be more emphasis on a treatment program that uses both psychoactive drugs and other types of therapy in combination. There seems to be less treatment by private physicians and fewer cases where the patient is simply evaluated and sent off to another treatment facility. Larger psychiatric facilities often have additional programs for specific types of patients (i.e., adolescents, drug addicts, autistic children, etc.) and research facilities. There is considerable variation in how long a patient stays in this type of center. Some patients stay for as long as a year if they can afford to do so.

General hospitals sometimes offer services other than in-patient care. Common services are emergency psychiatric treatment, out-patient individual or group therapy for a few hours per week, day treatment programs, night hospitalization, and special teams. An emergency psychiatric service is usually located within the general emergency facilities of the hospital. It provides assistance both to individuals who come primarily for psychiatric reasons and to those whose primary complaint is a physical illness or injury. The services usually offered are evaluation, crisis intervention, referral to other community agencies, and referral to the inpatient or out-patient facility of the hospital. Some emergency units also have a twenty-four-hour telephone service which people may call for help. Through telephone communication, a person may be given assistance with such problems as the desire to commit suicide, a family crisis, or simply the need to talk to someone who might be understanding.

Out-patient individual or group therapy for a few hours per week is usually available both to patients who have received in-patient treatment and to those who have been referred by the emergency psychiatric service. This division of a general hospital's psychiatric program may offer a considerable variety of treatment, such as monthly meetings of doctor and patient to determine if the patient needs any change in his use of psychoactive drugs, family therapy, marriage counseling, and special problem groups, such as groups for parents of drug addicts or persons with work-related difficulties, and social groups for previously hospitalized patients.

Similarly, day treatment programs are usually available to former in-patients and to persons referred by the emergency psychiatric service. The actual setting of this program is often outside the general hospital. It may, for example, be located in the basement of a church, in a store front, or in a settlement house. Participants in the program usually come at nine in the morning and stay until three or four o'clock in the afternoon. Involvement in the program is usually limited to approximately three months.

Night hospitalization refers to a program wherein the patient is involved in his usual activities in the community during the day but spends his evenings and sleeps at the treatment center at night. This program may be oriented to one of two goals. It may be designed to help a patient move out of the hospital. When the program has this orientation, it is very similar to a halfway house program. The patient is provided with room and board while he begins once again to participate in community activities. Patients in the program usually meet for an hour or two several evenings each week. In these meetings patients are encouraged to talk about how they are adjusting to life outside the hospital. They are able to get help with current problems, and they provide reassurance and support for each other. The other purpose of a night hospitalization program is to offer intensive treatment for people who either cannot give up their responsibilities in the community or who should not because fulfilling these responsibilities provides the core of their identity. An example of the former is a mother with four preschool children; an example of the latter is a bank manager whose job literally is his entire life. Patients who are involved in a night hospital program for intensive treatment are the kind of people who can perform their usual responsibilities but need distance from these responsibilities or massive support while developing other facets of the self.

Special teams supported by general hospitals are usually made up of mental health workers with a variety of professional backgrounds. For example, they may include a physician, a nurse, a dietician, a social worker, and an activities therapist. Special teams are developed to deal with a particular problem that is best handled in the community rather than by bringing people into the hospital setting. For example, a special team may be developed to work in a "welfare hotel." These hotels are the permanent residence of people, usually elderly, whose major form of financial support is welfare payments. The team may be invited to work in the hotel by some sort of tenant association, or the team may ask the tenant association if they may come into the hotel to assist the residents. The purpose of the team is to help the residents with whatever medical, social, or psychological problems they may have. Diagnosis and treatment for minor illnesses may be provided in a small clinic located in the hotel. Individuals with chronic deseases may be evaluated periodically. The residents are helped to develop group social activities. Isolated residents may be encouraged to join in the life of the hotel. Residents are sometimes given advice about and assistance in dealing with complex institutions in the community. There may be a program for treatment of psychosocial dysfunction. The special team maintains a close liaison with the general hospital. Usually arrangements are made for out-patient services for residents who need this kind of help.

Another type of special team may be assigned to a local, city-run day care center for preschool children. The team assesses the health and well-being of the children, offering advice to the staff members of the center about ways of dealing with specific difficulties. Parents are often invited to participate in the program. The special team, for example, may be available for individual conferences with parents and for group meetings to discuss problems in child rearing.

Other Facilities

This is a miscellaneous category which includes a variety of different types of centers or programs. One example is a day treatment center for select patients which is supported by a psychoanalytic training institute. In this type of center, as an illustration, young adult schizophrenic patients may be encouraged to participate in a program that combines verbal and activities therapy. There are also facilities, not associated with any hospital, that have programs for discharged psychiatric patients. Some of these programs have one major focus, such as the development of work habits. Others are more generalized, offering both learning experiences in many areas and a social-recreational program. These non-hospital-related facilities also usually offer advice, assistance, and support with regard to problems participants may face in the wider community. Prescriptions for psychoactive drugs, however, are usually not available. Other types of services that fall into this category are social-recreational programs for formerly hospitalized psychiatric patients sponsored, for example, by a church group or a "Y." The sponsoring organization may offer such programs as arts and crafts instruction, planned trips, social coffee hours, and holiday parties.

The facilities described above are probably not a complete listing of all of the programs concerned with helping psychiatric patients. We have provided here only a brief survey to give the beginning activities therapist some idea of the various types of psychiatric facilities.

EXAMPLES OF WHAT HAPPENS ON THE WARD OR IN A ONE-UNIT CENTER

The purpose of this section is to orient the beginning activities therapist to typical programs that she might encounter. These are, again, just examples; each treatment unit has its own special way of organizing itself. The examples given are only for programs that actively make use of activities therapy.

A Day Treatment Center

In the day treatment center to be described, the patients and staff arrive around nine o'clock in the morning. They spend the first half hour in the general meeting room having coffee and "warming up" for the day ahead. At 9:30 they divide into two groups for a meeting. There are approximately twelve patients in each group and three staff members. The first part of the meeting (about half an hour) is devoted to talking about any problems the patients have encountered since they left the center the previous afternoon. The next two hours are devoted to deciding on and carrying out an activity or continuing with an on-going activity. These groups are devoted to development of facets of the private self. Patients and staff bring their lunch, which is eaten in small informal groups in various parts of the center.

After lunch, there is a free recreation period with a gym available for active sports and games. The next hour and a half are devoted to individual or group treatment. Experiences are designed to develop basic skills and facets of the public self. Although it generally appears to be only loosely organized, this is a well-planned part of the program. It is fluid and ever-changing. Different kinds of activities groups and one-to-one interactions are formed and dissolved depending on the current needs of each patient. Patients and staff members plan activities together. Patients very quickly learn what experiences can be of help to them. And with intimate knowledge of each other's areas of difficulties, they are in a position to select appropriate activities. One therapist is usually included in each group or one-to-one interaction. But, at times, a therapist is not needed or her presence is not desirable.

From 3:30 to 4:00 P.M. all members of the community, patients and staff members, come together for a "community meeting." A community meeting is a common feature of many different kinds of treatment centers and programs. Although there are variations, a community meeting usually involves discussion of current problems of the unit, interpersonal difficulties, and future plans or projects. It is a meeting to enhance the living and working together of the community. This meeting is not designed to be a treatment group. Learning can and does occur, but the main purpose of the community meeting is to attend to the business of the community. After the community meeting, the patients go home. Staff members usually meet together for a half hour or so to talk about what happened during the day, problems that certain patients may be having, staff members' difficulties in relating to each other or patients, and to make plans for the next day. Patients are free to attend this meeting if they want to do so.

Every Friday, the two small morning groups spend part of their meeting time talking about what each group member has learned or accomplished that week. There is discussion of each patient's future plans, in terms of both how he is going to make use of the day treatment center in the coming weeks and what he is going to do after he leaves the program.

When a person first comes to the day treatment center, he is met by one staff member and patient from the morning group to which he has been assigned. After a brief orientation, he immediately joins in the program. Sometime during the first three days, he participates in an evaluation session or sessions with the staff member who greeted him on the first morning. On the fourth day of a patient's participation in the program, he and the therapist talk with the morning group about the patient's areas of difficulty and the goals the patient has set for his involvement in the program. Other group members give the patient feedback about what they see as his problem areas and the appropriateness of his goals. Everyone tries to be supportive of the patient and offer him encouragement.

The staff member who helps a patient to identify problem areas becomes the patient's "primary therapist." A primary therapist coordinates the patient's treatment program, encourages involvement in appropriate learning experiences, and acts as the patient's counselor and guide while he is at the treatment center. A patient is urged to turn to his primary therapist for whatever aid or assistance he may need.

A patient usually comes to the day treatment center for three months. The target date for leaving is established when the patient first comes to the center. If a patient wishes to leave earlier or to continue treatment for a longer period of time, he is encouraged to discuss this with his small morning group. They give the patient feedback about his decision and help him decide if this is the best course of action. Patients are usually strongly discouraged from staying in the program longer than three months. However, there are a few patients who can truly benefit from a slightly longer period of treatment. These patients are urged to take advantage of the additional time for learning.

A Ward of a Decentralized State Hospital

There are approximately forty patients on this hypothetical ward, a daytime staff of four, an evening staff of two, and one staff member on the ward at night. In addition to the bedrooms, the ward has a dining room, a kitchen, a dayroom, an arts and crafts room, a room for small group meetings, and office space.

Patients get up around seven o'clock, dress, and clean up their bedrooms. Breakfast is at eight o'clock. It is brought to the ward and served by people from the general kitchen in the building. There is a community meeting at nine o'clock. The meeting is similar to the one described for the day treatment center. In addition, however, there is discussion about what went on during the previous evening and night. Someone reads aloud the notes left by the night staff member. Decisions about, for example, whether a patient is ready for a home visit or able to go to the canteen alone are also made at this meeting.

After the community meeting, the patients and staff break up into four small groups. These groups are called "daily living groups." Each group has a general assignment: preparing lunch, care of the ward, ward improvement, or fund raising. These assignments are usually rotated every week. Daily living group members decide how they want to carry out their assignment within the limits of the ward situation. For example, the lunch group can order food from the kitchen or get permission from the community to buy special supplies from the local grocery store. They might make a cake to celebrate someone's birthday or plan a holiday meal. The group works within a budget, plans, prepares, and serves the lunch, and cleans up the kitchen. The ward care group takes responsibility for cleaning the ward plus special cleaning projects such as waxing the floors or washing the windows. They purchase or order items for the ward, take care of the bulletin board, make holiday decorations, and so forth. The ward improvement group is responsible for small repairs on the ward and major tasks such as making bookcases, painting the bathroom, and sewing curtains. They work within a budget provided by the hospital and use money raised by the fund-raising group. The group may decide on a project themselves, or a suggestion may be made by someone outside the group. In either case, the plan for the project has to be approved at a community meeting. The fund-raising group is responsible for raising money for the use of the ward. In addition to the mentioned uses of ward money, it is also spent for such things as trips into the community, delivery of the newspaper, an impromptu evening pizza party, and loans to patients. The fund-raising group plans its own projects. They might make macramé belts to be sold to a handcraft shop in the community, bake cupcakes to sell to another ward in the evening, set up a building-wide lottery, or sell tickets for a concert given by a local rock group which they have invited to the hospital.

The daily living groups are designed to teach basic skills, work habits, some aspects of activities of daily living, and to develop facets of the private self. Work on the task is interrupted any time a group member, staff or patient, feels that discussion of what is happening in the group would be useful. The discussion may be about how someone is feeling or acting, a conflict between two members, why no one seems interested in the task, *how* you wash a window, and the like. Usually toward the end of each daily living group meeting, group members take time out to talk about what happened in the group that day. They identify useful, need-satisfying behavior that occurred in the group and ways of behaving that could be improved upon. Group members give feedback to each other, offer suggestions, and provide encouragement. The pressure of the task is kept fairly low, so that important learning can take place. However, there is a general expectation that the task will be accomplished.

After an hour lunch period, a majority of the patients leave the ward to participate in hospital-wide activities. These may include such activities as working in the patient-run canteen or at another hospital job, going to a class to prepare for taking a high school equivalency examination, learning to cook or sew in the homemaking program, or taking typing lessons. Special staff members who are not attached to any wards are responsible for the hospital-wide program. However, they maintain a close liaison with the ward, coming to the community meetings to report on the progress of ward patients who are in the programs and helping patients determine if they are ready for hospital-wide programs.

Patients who are not ready to participate in more advanced activities remain on the ward. Staff members help these patients learn such things as task skills, simple activities of daily living, and basic group-interaction skills. Patients who have acquired the skills that are learned through hospital-wide activities go out into the community to facilitate further learning and readjustment to the community. These are patients who are almost ready to leave the hospital. Some patients hold part-time jobs; others may go home to spend time with their children; still others take courses in the local junior college, look for a job, or go shopping. When a patient is to continue treatment in a satellite center, he may spend several afternoons visiting the center prior to becoming a full-time member.

Everyone, except patients who have gone out into the community, is usually back on the ward by 3:30. Coffee has been made by patients who stayed on the ward. There is a half hour informal gathering in the day room. If anyone feels the need for a meeting of his small group, group members take their coffee to a smaller room. A meeting may be called because one of the group members has something he wants to talk about, or there may be unfinished business from the morning meeting.

Dinner is at five o'clock. The evening and weekend are devoted primarily to recreation. There is an effort on everyone's part to use the time in a need-satisfying manner. The arts and crafts room and the kitchen are open. Patients are encouraged to organize activities such as a Ping-Pong tournament, charades, or an old-fashioned songfest. More long-term activities are also encouraged; for example, patients may plan and organize an all-building bazaar or prepare skits for a hospital-wide variety show. There may be group trips into the community for a movie or a spaghetti dinner. A patient center on the grounds of the hospital provides an opportunity for patients to participate in sports and table games, visit the "coffee house," browse in the library, talk with friends in the lounge, and join in various hobby groups organized by volunteers. The patient center is run jointly by a permanent group of staff members and patients from various wards.

Orientation to the program, evaluation, discussion of progress, procedures for leaving the hospital, and the role of the primary therapist are similar to those outlined for the day treatment center. However, the target date for leaving the hospital is usually one to two months. There is also more concern with medication. In the day treatment center, either patients need no medication or the process of finding the right drug and dosage has been completed. This process usually has to be started on the ward. This can be a difficult time for patients; the side effects of many psychoactive drugs are uncomfortable and some patients do not like the idea of taking any type of drug. Patients are given support during this trying time, and concessions are made regarding the ward norm of active participation in the activities.

Social visiting is encouraged in the evenings and on weekends. Patients are urged to spend the weekend or at least part of it visiting friends or family or both. Visitors are welcome on the ward, either to join in the recreational activities or to have a private chat with the patient. Staff members are available to help with any difficulty in patients and visitors relating to each other. For example, a patient may need help in explaining how he thinks his family may be of assistance to him, or a friend may have questions about the patient's treatment that the patient is not able to answer. Visiting is discouraged on weekdays because it is felt that this is the time for patients to be involved in the work of treatment.

A Large Unit of a General Hospital

This large psychiatric unit of a general hospital is housed in a separate building. There are approximately two hundred patients living on ten wards. The activities therapy department is assigned two floors. They have a gym, a prevocational unit, specialized shops (i.e., woodworking, ceramics, jewelry, etc.), a kitchen, a dining area, general arts and crafts rooms, and small meeting rooms.

Patients get up about seven o'clock, dress, clean up their rooms, and eat breakfast at eight o'clock. All meals are served in a patient-staff cafeteria. There is a community meeting on each ward at nine o'clock. At ten o'clock patients from all the wards disperse to various programs offered by the activities therapy department. Lunch is served from 12:00 to 1:30.

Patients then return to the ward for a one-hour verbal group therapy meeting. This meeting is different from a community meeting in that individual, personal problems are discussed in considerable depth. In a community meeting, a patient's individual difficulties are discussed only if they affect the overall functioning of the ward. For example, in a community meeting, it might be suggested that everyone keep all of his valued possessions in his locker until Harriet learns to stop taking things that do not belong to her. In the verbal group therapy meeting, the group would help Harriet consider the reasons for her stealing and suggest better ways of satisfying needs. Verbal group therapy differs from activities group therapy. In an activities therapy group, a patient's difficulty in functioning is focused upon when the problem is apparent in the context of the activity. Discussion is usually confined to what just happened and what the patient can do about it within the context of the immediate situation. In verbal group therapy, problem areas are explored relative to how they affect a patient's interactions in a number of different situations, both in the hospital and prior to hospitalization. The recent past, within the last couple of months or the last two years, is talked about, but not historical events such as, "When I was four years old . . ." To illustrate, in an activities therapy group, Luther may be asked how he felt just before he grabbed the broom out of Edith's hands. He says that he cannot stand to see someone doing a sloppy job. The group then helps him to think about other ways that he might have dealt both with his feelings and with the situation. He is then encouraged to approach Edith again and to "replay" the incident. In verbal group therapy, Luther may raise the point that he cannot tolerate imperfection in himself or others. He has very high standards, which he feels that everyone should meet. Luther may be asked to talk about what "being imperfect" means to him, what would happen if he did not live up to his high standards, what kind of imperfections particularly bother him, and so forth. The group tries to help Luther understand his purpose in maintaining high standards, and how this interferes with his need satisfaction. Practical actions that Luther might take to learn to live with imperfection are identified. Incidents that occurred in the activities therapy program may be used as a point of departure for discussion in verbal group therapy. Ideas, feelings, and problem areas discussed in verbal group therapy may help to clarify what a patient needs to give attention to in activities therapy.

After group therapy, patients either return to activities therapy or go out into the community to practice application of newly acquired skills. This time for practice in the community is similar to what is done in the ward of the state hospital described previously. Dinner is from 5:00 to 6:30. The activities therapy program continues until nine o'clock.

Two activities therapists are assigned to each ward. They participate in the ward's daily community meeting, verbal group therapy, and staff meetings. Each therapist acts as the primary activities therapist for half the patients on the ward. Beyond these responsibilities, the therapists devote their time to working in the activities therapy program.

The activities therapy department provides both treatment and recreational opportunities. The recreational part of the program is different from helping someone learn how to make use of free time. That is treatment. The kind of recreation referred to here is to have fun. It is not designed for learning but to have a good time, given one's assets and limitations. In other words, no one is asking the patient to examine his ideas or feelings or try behaving in a different way. Recreation is a relief from treatment.

The kinds of experiences offered by the activities therapy department are extensive. Some examples are modern and folk dancing, movement groups, listening to music, piano and guitar lessons, basketball, volleyball, baseball, swimming, exercise groups, play reading, arts and crafts, hospital and community job placement, work groups, sheltered workshop experiences, cooking, photography, activities of daily living experiences, a mural painting group, and so on. The types of activities available are ever-changing, depending on the needs and interests of the patients, the skills of the activities therapy staff, and the type of volunteers available. As mentioned, some of these activities are designed for treatment, others are purely recreational in nature. (Volunteers participate only in recreational activities.) Activities may take place in groups or in one-to-one interactions.

Upon admission to the hospital, the patient participates in evaluation with the therapist who will be his primary activities therapist. For the first few days, the patient goes only to recreational activities. When the patient and therapist have decided what the patient needs to learn, a weekly schedule is prepared. The therapist, knowing the purpose of all the experiences currently available in the activities therapy department, helps the patient decide what activities will enhance his learning. Treatment-oriented activities are interspersed with recreational activities to give a work-play balance to each day. The schedule includes periods for personal chores such as doing one's laundry and free time periods if this is desirable for the patient's growth. Some patients in the hospital participate in individual verbal psychotherapy. This is also included in the schedule. A patient may or may not participate in individual activities therapy with his primary therapist. The decision depends on his learning needs and on the experiences available in the activities therapy department. The patient and therapist periodically review the patient's progress, making changes in his activities schedule as needed.

There are several all-hospital groups in this treatment center. These groups are initiated by patients; staff members are sometimes invited to participate. One of the more active groups is patient government. A representative from each ward meets twice a week to talk about current problems and issues that affect the whole hospital. The areas in which the patient government is able to make decisions have been carefully worked out with the therapeutic staff and hospital administration. For example, they have the power to make rules regarding dress and conduct in public areas. They do not have a final say on visiting hours. However, the recommendations of the patient government are sought on many decisions that the staff must make.

There is a hospital-wide committee to plan for special events, such as what to do to commemorate Martin Luther King's birthday and would the patients and staff be interested in a lecture-demonstration about acupuncture. *Ad hoc* groups are formed to deal with temporary matters. For example, there may be a group formed to revise the "Patient Orientation Booklet," or several patients may get together to see if anything can be done about the dilapidated tables in the cafeteria. There are usually one or more active ethnic groups. The purpose of these groups may be to maintain group members' ethnic identity, to discuss problems and interests unique to the group, to deal actively with discrimination in the hospital, or a combination of these goals.

SUMMARY

Of necessity, many details of the way a treatment center is organized and goes about its daily work have been omitted in the above examples. This chapter was intended to give a flavor of what an activities therapist might find in a treatment center. The descriptions given here have presented an overview of the structure or framework for patient care. The actual evaluation and treatment process were simply mentioned rather than examined in detail. The following chapters are devoted to discussion of these processes, which are central to the work of an activities therapist.

SUGGESTED READING

Binderman, A., and Spiegel, A. *Perspective in Community Mental Health.* Chicago: Aldine Publishing Company, 1969.

Kramer, Bernard. *Day Hospital.* New York: Grune & Stratton, 1962.

Parnud, Howard. *Crisis Intervention.* New York: Family Service Association of America, 1965.

Roberts, L., Halleck, S., and Loch, M. *Community Psychiatry.* Garden City, N.Y.: Doubleday & Company, 1969.

Tulipan, A., and Heyder, D. *Outpatient Psychiatry in the 1970's.* New York: Brummer/Mozel Publishers, 1970.

Whittington, H. G. *Psychiatry in the American Community.* New York: International Universities Press, 1966.

Whittington, H. G. *Development of an Urban Mental Health Center.* Springfield, Ill.: Charles C. Thomas, 1971.

CHAPTER 6

EVALUATION

Evaluation is the process of determining what the patient is able to do and what he is not able to do. The process of evaluation should not be confused with diagnosis. Diagnosis involves assigning a medical label, such as schizophrenia or manic-depression, as a way of identifying the nature of the patient's psychosocial dysfunction. Activities therapists may contribute to diagnosis by sharing information about a patient with a physician. However, activities therapists do not make diagnoses; they evaluate.

Evaluation findings are used by the patient and therapist as the basis for planning treatment. Evaluation is a collaborative process between patient and therapist. That is, the patient and therapist work together to identify the patient's assets and limitations. Thus, the patient should be aware that he is being evaluated, what he is being evaluated for, and what he is expected to do during the evaluation process. Evaluative findings are shared with the patient. Ideally, the evaluative process is designed to help the patient identify his own problems in living. Self-discovery of problem areas is often more meaningful to a patient than having someone else tell him what his problems are.

THE PROCESS IN GENERAL

There are two kinds of evaluation: initial and periodic. Initial evaluation is assessment of the patient's difficulties prior to beginning treatment. It may be total or partial. *Total* initial evaluation is assessment of all possible areas of dysfunction; *partial* initial evaluation is assessment of only some possible areas of dysfunction. For example, in partial initial evaluation, the patient and therapist may first explore the patient's ability to engage in simple tasks and to function adequately in a group. At a later time, during the treatment process, difficulties in activities of daily living and work might be explored. All of these areas (and others) would be assessed at the same time in a total initial evaluation procedure. Whether an initial evaluation should be total or partial is a decision that the therapist must make. The only guideline suggested here is that it is probably best to involve patients who appear to have considerable difficulty doing almost anything in a partial evaluation. Patients who appear to have less difficulty in functioning can usually participate in a total initial evaluation.

Periodic evaluation is assessment of the patient's progress or lack of progress during the course of treatment. It is a formal, regular part of the treatment process. It is *formal* in the sense that time is specifically set aside to look at what improvements the patient may or may not have experienced. The therapist and patient sit down together to discuss what the patient is able to do now that he was not able to do at the time of the initial evaluation or the last periodic evaluation. All identified areas of dysfunction are explored. Periodic evaluations are *regular* in the sense that they occur at specific predetermined times during treatment. Ideally, periodic evaluation occurs once every week. Once a month is probably the longest time that should elapse between periodic evaluations. Because periodic evaluation is an integral part of the treatment process, it will be discussed at greater length in Chapter 7.

An evaluation procedure can be broken down into three steps: observation, interpretation, and validation. *Observation* is noting what the patient says and what he does, or reading what he has written. It is taking note of "raw behavior" as opposed to ascribing meaning to a particular event. For example, noting that a patient continually requests assistance and often asks the therapist if he is doing an assigned task the right way is observation. Saying that a patient is dependent is not observation; it is interpretation. It is often useful to take notes during observation. Patients rarely object to this if they are told how the notes will be used and why note-taking enhances the evaluation process. Patients sometimes feel more comfortable if they are assured that they may read the notes after the evaluation procedure is over. If the therapist decides not to take notes, observations should be written down as soon as possible after an evaluation procedure. The greater the lapse of time between observation and recording, the more likely it is that some observations will be forgotten.

The next step in evaluation is interpretation. *Interpretation* is assigning meaning to what has been observed. It is the process of using observed data to determine what the patient is and is not able to do. For example, Angela spends all her time taking care of her family's needs, and reports that she feels guilty about taking time to do things she particularly enjoys. From these observations, the therapist might conclude that Angela has a value system that is interfering with her need satisfaction. This is an interpretation.

The third step in evaluation is validation. *Validation* is the process of seeking confirmation regarding the accuracy of an interpretation. The best source for confirmation is the patient. This is one of the reasons why it is suggested that the therapist share evaluation findings with the patient. Occasionally, however, a patient is not ready to admit that he is having difficulty in a particular area. Thus, at times, validation may also be sought from the patient's family, fellow therapists, or other staff members. Seeking validation should not be seen as a contest of finding out who is right and who is wrong. Rather, it is a sharing of opinions and ideas.

Evaluation should take place as soon as possible after the patient is admitted to the treatment center. The only exception is when the patient has symptoms that can often be diminished by the use of therapeutic drugs. In such a case, it is sometimes better to wait until medication has had at least some effect. By waiting, the therapist is likely to get a more accurate picture of the patient's problem areas. In addition, the patient is usually much more able to cooperate in the evaluation process. The period set aside for initial evaluation is relatively short, preferably not more than one week. Treatment can thus be initiated without undue delay. A short initial evaluation period often means that some desired information is not available. However, no matter how long a period is set aside for evaluation, additional information is usually wanted. Initial evaluations are always tentative and subject to change. This is one of the reasons that periodic evaluations are part of the treatment process.

Evaluation should be as efficient as possible. When several people are to be involved in evaluating the same patient, the evaluation is planned so that there is minimal overlap in the information each person requests of the patient. This is most easily accomplished if each person on the evaluation team knows what information each team member usually requests of a patient. It is a waste of both staff and patient time for many staff members to investigate the same area. Thus, for example, if the nurse usually looks for problems in activities of daily living, there is no reason for the occupational therapist to evaluate this area as well.

A therapist sometimes questions whether she should read the reports of other staff members before or after making her own evaluation of the patient. The advantage of reading reports *before* evaluation is that the therapist has some clues about the patient's difficulties. The disadvantage is the possibility of paying more attention to the written report than to what the patient is actually saying and doing during the evaluation procedure. The advantage of reading other staff members' reports *after* evaluating the patient is that the therapist is not biased by previous information. Thus, her report presents an independent point of view about the patient. The disadvantage is that the therapist knows nothing about the patient prior to the initial interview. It is probably best for the beginning therapist to try both methods before deciding which one is best for her.

The concept of "expected environment" is a significant part of the evaluation process. *Expected environment* refers to the anticipated life situation of the patient after treatment has ended. In determining the expected environment, the patient and therapist are concerned with such questions as: Where will the patient be living? With whom? What will be the patient's responsibilities in his home? Will the patient be working? What kind of job will he probably have? What types of avocational pursuits will be available for the patient? Identifying the expected environment in the initial evaluation helps both the patient and the therapist to set treatment goals and goal priorities. Naturally, the expected environment may change during treatment. Thus, it is discussed during each periodic evaluation.

The first meeting between patient and therapist is very important. Initial impressions are formed quickly and are often difficult to change, particularly if they are negative. To make this first meeting as successful as possible, the therapist attempts to find a place to talk with the patient that is relatively free from distractions. The therapist introduces herself and encourages the patient to do likewise. The therapist then explains briefly what activities therapy is all about, defining both her role and the role of the patient in evaluation and treatment. Explanation is given at a level that the patient seems to be able to understand. (It is sometimes difficult to determine whether the patient in fact understands what the therapist is saying; one indication is whether he asks questions that are related to the information that has been presented.) Also, one does not overwhelm the patient with information. This can be confusing, with the result that the patient may remember little of what has been said. The patient is encouraged to ask questions or to express any of his immediate concerns. Answers to questions are as honest and forthright as possible. The therapist should never be afraid to say, "I don't know." Reassurance is given, but not the false, hearty type. That is, the therapist says she believes she can help the patient if he is willing to help himself. She never says she is sure treatment will eliminate all of the patient's difficulties, or that treatment is an easy, unpainful process. Treatment is not fun and games; it is hard work for both the patient and therapist. Time is always left for casual conversation if the patient is able to tolerate this type of interaction. The therapist indicates her concern for the patient as an individual with unique qualities. The patient is never made to feel that evaluation is an impersonal, assembly-line procedure. It is a personal assessment in which the patient is intimately involved. After the first meeting, the therapist and patient may begin evaluation immediately, or the therapist may make an appointment to begin evaluation in the immediate future. When questionnaires are part of the evaluative procedure, they may be given to the patient to fill out before the first evaluation session.

The evaluation techniques most typically used in activities therapy are observation, structured observation, interview, and questionnaires. As used here, *observation* refers to noting a patient's usual patterns of behavior. For example, the therapist notes whether or not the patient is generally appropriately dressed. No specially designed situation is required to make this observation. Conversely, *structured observation* involves setting up a specific situation and asking the patient to participate in the situation, for example, requesting that the patient be involved in planning a group project or asking the patient to type a letter. An *interview* is a one-to-one discussion with the patient. It is designed to get specific information. An *interview schedule* is usually used to help the therapist obtain the desired information. Such a schedule typically consists of a list of questions or areas for discussion. A *questionnaire* is a written list of questions the patient is asked to answer as completely as possible. It may also include items the patient is supposed to check or circle. When a patient is asked to fill out a questionnaire, the therapist and patient usually discuss the completed questionnaire together. This is perhaps the best procedure if a questionnaire is used. It makes filling out the questionnaire a less impersonal process, and clarifies any misconceptions the therapist might have regarding the information the patient is trying to communicate. Also, some patients find it difficult to complete a questionnaire without some assistance.

ASSESSMENT OF ASSETS AND LIMITATIONS

The following discussion is outlined according to suggested ways of evaluating each facet of man. This technique is in a sense artificial, because in the actual evaluation of a patient, many areas may be assessed at the same time. However, for the sake of clarity and simplicity, we shall here discuss each area in isolation.

The methods for evaluation outlined below are only suggestions. Other methods may be more appropriate for a particular center because of the unique needs or characteristics of the patient population. The evaluation suggested may seem rather lengthy and complex, especially for a short-term treatment center. Thus, the therapist may decide to use only parts of the evaluation or to evaluate in a less detailed manner. A complete "Activities Therapy Evaluation Questionnaire" is not presented here. The following discussion of evaluation is based on the use of structured interviews. However, from the suggested interview schedules and other forms presented, the therapist may wish to design a questionnaire.

There is some general information the therapist will want to know as soon as possible:

> Patient's name and address, marital status, and age.
> Years of schooling completed.
> Education orientation (vocational, commercial, or college preparatory program in high school; college major).
> Other education (trade school, training in armed services, business college, etc.).
> With whom the patient is living currently, or was living prior to hospitalization.
> Why the patient is seeking treatment.

At some point in the initial evaluation (usually near the end), the therapist seeks the following information from the patient:

> What do you consider to be your outstanding abilities, talents, and strong points?
> What do you want to change about yourself?
> What do you see yourself doing six months from now?
> A year from now? Five years from now?

Basic Skills

Task Skills. Task skill, as previously defined, is the ability to carry out an activity that requires the use of various tools and materials and the completion of several steps. It is concerned primarily with manipulation and use of the nonhuman environment. Assessment of this area usually occurs in the initial evaluation. It is accomplished by using structured observation; the patient is asked to complete a task that has the characteristics outlined above. In selecting an appropriate task, the therapist asks herself if a given activity could be completed successfully by a fully functioning individual who is similar to the patient in age and level of education. The patient's sex and cultural background are also taken into consideration in deciding on a task. Adequate directions (both verbal and written, if possible), tools, and materials necessary to complete the activity are made readily available. Assessment of task skills may be done in a one-to-one situation, or the therapist may evaluate several patients in this area at the same time. The therapist does not encourage interaction between patients if several patients are evaluated together. Such encouragement may interfere with a patient's ability to do the task.

The form on page 90 may be used by the therapist as an aid to observation. It is followed by a key for scoring. The key provides a description of each category on the form. A rating of 1 is given if the patient experiences considerable difficulty in a specific part of the task, whereas a rating of 4 indicates no difficulty with a given aspect of the task. The numbers 1 to 4 should be considered as being on a continuum. Thus, for example, a patient may be given a rating of 2 if he is so hyperactive that he has trouble carrying out the task. He may be given a rating of 1 if he is so hyperactive that he is unable to complete the task. Another way of looking at the 1-to-4 continuum is as follows:

1 = exhibits maladaptive behavior most of the time.
2 = exhibits maladaptive behavior some of the time.
3 = exhibits maladaptive behavior occasionally.
4 = exhibits no evidence of maladaptive behavior.

It is suggested that the Survey of Task Skills on page 90 be used in the following way: A rating of 1 to 4 is given to indicate placement of the patient on the continuum of described behavior. The number is en-

Survey of Task Skills [1]

Behavior	Comments	Present	Future
Coordination Bizarre behavior Hyperactivity Hypoactivity Reliability Engagement Concentration Directions Activity neatness Attention to detail Problem solving Organization of task			

[1] This survey and key for scoring are adapted from Gail and Jay Fidler, *Occupational Therapy: A Communication Process in Psychiatry,* New York: Macmillan Company, 1963.

Key for Survey of Task Skills

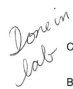

Coordination
    1 = Moves in a clumsy manner, has difficulty manipulating tools and materials
    4 = Is able to engage in activities that require both fine and gross movements
Bizarre behavior
    1 = Stereotyped activities (rocking, playing with hands, repetitive statements), appears
        to be talking to self, preoccupation with own thoughts, etc.
    4 = Absence of above
Hyperactivity
    1 = Accelerated in speech and/or action
    4 = Speaks and acts at normal pace
Hypoactivity
    1 = Retarded in speech and/or action
    4 = Speaks and acts at normal pace
Reliability
    1 = Cannot be depended on to carry out a given activity; inappropriate use of tools and
        materials
    4 = Can be depended on to perform in an acceptable manner
Engagement
    1 = Does not engage in activity
    4 = Readily engages in activity without encouragement
Concentration
    1 = Readily loses interest in a given task
    4 = Works at a given task with sustained interest and attention
Directions
    1 = Unable to carry out simple demonstrated, oral, and/or written directions
    4 = Readily carries out relatively complex demonstrated, oral, and written directions
Activity neatness
    1 = Performs activities in a sloppy, careless manner
    4 = Performs activities in a neat, orderly manner
Attention to detail
    1 = Overly concise to the point that it interferes with performance
    4 = Attends to detail according to the demands of the given activity

Problem solving
   1 = Activity behavior is disrupted when confronted with problems that arise in the context
       of an activity; no attempt is made to solve them
   4 = Identifies and solves problems which arise in the performance of an activity; uses
       resources in an appropriate manner
Organization of task
   1 = Unable to organize an activity effectively even when tools, materials, and directions
       are available
   4 = Organizes a task in a logical and efficient manner

tered in the "Present" column. The "Comments" column is used to record specific things the patient did or said which led the therapist to assign the number. For example, "asked for help whenever he encountered a simple problem" or "no attempt at overt trial and error when fitting pieces together" might be entered in the "Comments" column after problem solving. Entries in this column are as specific as possible. This is the place for the "raw behavior" mentioned in the first part of this chapter. When the therapist is uncertain as to what number to assign a particular aspect of task skill, it can be left blank and inserted at a later time.

The "Future" column is tentatively completed at the time of the initial evaluation. A rating of 1 to 4 is assigned based on the patient's anticipated expected environment. The guiding question is what degree of task skill the patient will need to get along in his expected environment. As mentioned, expected environment is always tentative at the beginning of treatment. Its usefulness here is to determine whether or not the patient needs help in this area. For example, the patient who is planning on returning to a job where he is told exactly what to do and how to do it is going to need less skill in problem solving than the patient who is self-employed. A great difference between numbers in the "Present" column versus those in the "Future" column indicates considerable difficulty in the area of task skills. Little discrepancy indicates minimal difficulty.

After the patient has completed the evaluative task or has completed as much as he can, the therapist discusses the task with the patient. The Survey of Task Skills is often used as the basis for discussion. The therapist, after explaining the form and key, indicates what ratings she has assigned the patient in the "Present" column. Validation is sought from the patient, and differences in points of view can be explored. This is also a good time to talk about the patient's expected future environment. It is often a good idea for the therapist and patient to fill out the "Future" column together at this time.

Group-Interaction Skills Survey

Type of Group	
Parallel Group	
Engages in some activity, but acts as if this is an individual task as opposed to a group activity	
Aware of others in the group	
Some verbal or nonverbal interaction with others	
Appears to be relatively comfortable in this situation	
Project Group	
Occasionally engages in the group activity, moving in and out according to his own whim	
Seeks some assistance from others	
Gives some assistance when directly asked to do so	
Egocentric-Cooperative Group	
Aware of group's goal relative to the task	
Aware of group norms	
Acts as if he belongs in the group	
Willing to participate	
Meets esteem needs of others	
Able to get others to meet his esteem needs	
Recognizes rights of others	
Not overly competitive	
Cooperative Group	
Makes own wishes, desires, and needs known	
Participates in group activity but seems concerned primarily with his own needs and needs of others	
Able to meet needs other than esteem needs	
Tends to be most responsive to group members who are similar to him in some way	
Mature Group	
Responsive to all group members	
Takes a variety of task roles	
Takes a variety of social-emotional roles	
Able to share leadership	
Promotes a good balance between task accomplishment and satisfaction of group members' needs	

Adaptive Skill

Group-Interaction Skills. Group interaction, as previously defined, is the ability to be a productive member of a variety of small groups. Like assessment of task skills, assessment of group interaction is usually a part of the initial evaluation. One way to evaluate for this area is through structured observation. The situation may be designed as follows: Five to seven new patients are requested to participate in an activity that requires collaborative interaction. The therapist selects the activity, but the patients are responsible for deciding exactly how they will carry out the activity. Necessary equipment and materials are provided or made readily available. The therapist does not participate in the group. She

let pt. simply go; simply observe

observes the group and only answers questions that are specifically directed to her.

The Group-Interaction Skills Survey above may be used as an aid in observing and determining a patient's level of group-interaction skill. The right-hand column is checked if the patient exhibits the behavior listed in the left-hand column. If a patient exhibits all the behavior listed under a particular type of group, it is fairly safe to say that he would be able to participate in that kind of group in a variety of situations. When a patient does not exhibit all the behavior listed under a particular kind of group, he either has passed beyond that stage of skill development or has not yet completely mastered that level of group-interaction skill.

After the group has finished the evaluative activity, the therapist talks with each patient individually. Again, it is often useful to use the survey as a way of structuring the interview. The patient is shown his survey form already checked. The therapist tells the patient why certain behaviors were checked and others were not. The patient is then encouraged to express his opinion about his behavior in the group and whether this behavior is typical of his participation in other group situations. Discrepancies between the therapist's observations of him and the patient's observations of himself are then discussed. Hopefully, some agreement can be reached. During this interview, the therapist and patient also discuss the patient's expected environment. If possible, they tentatively decide the level of group-interaction skill the patient is going to need for successful participation in this environment.

The Public Self

Activities of Daily Living. Activities of daily living refers to all those activities that are concerned with self care, communication, and travel. The Activities of Daily Living Survey below lists a number of activities of daily living. This list is probably not complete, nor is it suitable for every patient population. It is presented only as a sample of the type of form to use. The "Present" column is checked if the patient is able to perform the activity listed in the "Activity" column. The "Future" column is checked if the patient will need to be able to do the activity in his expected environment. It is also checked if the patient indicates that he would like to perform this activity in the future.

One way of assessing activities of daily living is to go over the survey

Activities of Daily Living Survey

Activity	Present	Future
Adequate hygiene		
Hair combed, appropriately styled		
Dress appropriate for age, current fashion, and occasion		
Clothes clean and ironed		
Plan nutritious diet		
Cook		
Shop for food		
Know what change to expect from clerk		
Plan a budget		
Change a bed		
Sweep and dust		
Wash and dry dishes		
Household tasks (hang curtains, change light bulb and fuse, take an appliance to be fixed, etc.)		
Shop for clothes		
Wash clothes		
Iron clothes		
Sew on a button		
Fix a ripped seam		
Make a hem		
Find a number in the telephone book		
Get a number from the telephone operator		
Make a telephone call to request information		
Make a telephone call to leave a message		
Take a telephone message		
Write a personal letter		
Write a business letter		
Fill out various forms		
Travel on a bus, subway, and train		
Read a timetable		
Buy and return a ticket		
Follow a road, subway, and bus route map		
Drive a car		

with the patient. This may be sufficient if the therapist is fairly sure that the patient is able to assess independently his capacities and limitations in this area. Many patients have trouble doing this. Also, people are often hesitant to say they have difficulty in doing such "simple" things. Thus, structured observation is sometimes required. This involves asking the patient to do the tasks listed on the survey. Only those activities that the patient is likely to need to be able to do are assessed. Ideally, this is done in the patient's expected environment, since this is a more real situation. If it is not possible to do this, a simulated situation in the treatment center may be used. Specific procedures for evaluation are so dependent on what is available in the center that they will not be listed here. The therapist must often be ingenious in devising situations that will allow her and the patient to gain sufficient information. If structured observation is used, the therapist discusses the survey with the patient after it has been completed. Differences in opinion are discussed and resolved if possible. The "Future" column is tentatively completed at this time.

Work.[2] Work is an individual's primary occupation or job. Assessment in this area usually involves both an interview and structured observation. Evaluation focuses on the patient's past work history, his present assets and limitations in the area of work, and his future work plans.

In the interview, the patient is asked to talk about all of his past work experience, beginning with the last job he held. As part of this discussion, the patient is asked to give:

Approximate dates of beginning and leaving each job.
Job title and specific tasks he was expected to perform.
Approximate salary.
Reasons for leaving each job.

The patient is also asked:

Which of the jobs he liked best and why.
What three jobs he feels would be most interesting to him at this time.
Whether he has any particular work skills (e.g., typing, operating a special kind of machine, telephone repair, keypunch operator, etc.).

If the patient has a job to which he wants to return or had a job in the not too distant past and wishes to get a similar job, evaluation is specific to that type of work. In other words, the patient is evaluated for his ability to perform in a specific kind of work situation. The patient and therapist discuss the job in order to determine what types of interactions

---

[2] This discussion of work evaluation has been influenced by Gail Fidler and the assessment procedure used in the Activities Therapy Department at Hillside Hospital, Queens Village, New York.

Child Care Survey

Activity	Present	Future
Demonstrates affection		
Cares for physical needs (food, clothes, etc.)		
Plays with a child		
Plans activities for a child		
Disciplines a child in a consistent manner		
Secures periodic physical, dental, and eye examinations		
Maintains a safe home		
Secures adequate baby-sitting facilities		
Shows concern about child's education		
Maintains adequate balance between freedom and control		
Communicates in a forthright manner (does not give double messages)		
Gives child appropriate responsibilities		
Aware of child's needs		

and task skills are necessary to perform the job successfully. They look at specific activities that must be performed as well as at the kinds of interpersonal relationships required. A written list of necessary behaviors is prepared by the therapist and patient. This is then used as a check sheet on which the patient's ability to perform the job is recorded.

Next, the therapist attempts to find a work situation in the treatment center, the community, or a sheltered workshop that is as similar as possible to the type of job for which the patient is to be evaluated. The patient works in the evaluative job situation for approximately three to five days. He is observed by the therapist periodically as well as by his supervisor on the job. At the end of this period, the patient, therapist and work supervisor go over the previously prepared list of required behavior. Each type of behavior is discussed to determine whether or not the patient is able to perform in that area.

The evaluation technique suggested above is oriented primarily to assessment for a paying job in the business world. Work evaluation for a homemaker is somewhat different. Many of the tasks listed on the Activities of Daily Living Survey are job responsibilities for the homemaker. That survey may therefore be used as a guide for assessing some of the skills required of a homemaker if the items not related to homemaking skill are deleted. The Child Care Survey above may be used as a guide for evaluation of the parent role if the homemaker is responsible for taking care of one or more children. Initially, the patient and therapist go over the two surveys, checking all of the pertinent tasks the homemaker is able to perform. When either the patient or the therapist is uncertain about the patient's actual ability to carry out a given task, a situation is designed so that the patient can test his ability. With regard to child care, the ideal procedure is to observe the patient caring for his children in his own home. When this is not possible, data may be obtained from the patient as well as from his children, spouse, or close friend or relative.

In evaluating a patient's ability to function in a school situation, the therapist is concerned about the patient's capacity to get along with fellow classmates and an authority-teacher and to attend to the task of studying. Ideally, evaluation in this area takes place in a school setting. When this is not feasible, information about the patient's capacity to interact with classmates may be obtained from observation of the patient in a group situation. Similarly, encouraging the patient to participate in a situation in which he is required to follow the directions of an authority figure may provide information about the patient's relationship to his teachers. The therapist and patient discuss the patient's school-related problems in an attempt to identify exactly what the patient's difficulties are. Why can he not manage to function in the school setting? There are times when a student is having trouble in school because of a "cognitive-perceptual-motor" problem. The cognitive-perceptual-motor area refers to the process of taking in and organizing sensory information and using this information as the basis for action. Evaluation for and treatment of cognitive-perceptual-motor problems will not be discussed in this book. This is a highly specialized and complex field, and the beginning activities therapist is not usually prepared to deal with problems in this area.

When a patient has not worked recently, or has never worked for any extended period of time, a different kind of work evaluation is required. This evaluation focuses on the patient's ability to function in a general work situation but not in a specific job. The Work Survey below may be used as a guide for evaluation. Participation in a sheltered workshop program or an on-going work group is the best situation for evaluating work habits. The suggested work group is similar to the kind of group used for the development of work skills. It is described on pages 141–158. Three to five days is usually sufficient time for evaluation. After this

Work Survey

Activities	
Alters behavior appropriately on the basis of constructive criticism	
Follows written, oral, and demonstrated directions	
Sustains attention to work tasks	
Organizes tasks relative to priority	
Performs tasks in a normal amount of time	
Works at increased speed when required	
Returns to work when interrupted	
Carries on appropriate conversation when working	
Interrupts work tasks and carries on appropriate conversation	
Completes forms	
Plans work period so that required amount of work is accomplished	
Comes to work on time	
Stays at work for required period of time	
Appears able to work a normal work day	
Evokes a pleasant response from others	
Follows the norms of the work setting	
Gives assistance willingly	
Takes direction from a work supervisor	
Requests only an appropriate amount of need satisfaction from the work supervisor	

period, the patient, therapist, and supervisor of the sheltered workshop or work group go over the Work Survey together. The patient's assets and limitations are noted.

Recreation. Recreation has been defined as activities carried out for the sake of personal enjoyment or pleasure. The Recreation Survey below may be used as a guide for evaluation. The activities listed should be considered as examples of possible recreational activities. The therapist may want to develop a new survey when she becomes better acquainted with the patient population with which she is working. The patient and therapist go over the survey together. The "Present" column is checked if the patient has recently engaged in the indicated activity; the "Future" column is checked if the patient would like to engage in the activity in the future. In talking with the patient, the therapist attempts to determine if the patient has participated in an activity relatively frequently or only occasionally. The letters F (frequently) and O (occasionally) are sometimes used in the "Present" column to indicate frequency. This is useful information, because it helps the patient and therapist decide whether the patient is spending his recreational time in a way that is truly satisfying to him. An individual sometimes engages in a recreational activity that he does not

Recreation Survey [3]

Activity	Present	Future	Activity	Present	Future
Swimming			Poetry		
Table games (poker, chess, bridge)			Going out to a restaurant or bar		
Photography			Political organizations		
Drama groups			Modern dancing		
Discussion groups			Sketching		
Choral groups			Painting		
Woodworking			Gymnastics		
Reading			Boxing		
Playing musical instrument			Wrestling		
Listening to music			Cooking		
Social dancing			Baseball		
Pool			Basketball		
Sewing			Football		
Bicycling			Tennis		
Movies			Golf		
Going to parties			Skiing		
Union activities			Sculpture		
Bowling			Electronics		
Lectures			Knitting		
Attending classes to learn how to do something			Calesthenics		
			Watching television		
			Casual conversation		
Gardening			Fixing things		
Shopping			PTA		
Church organizations			Volunteer work		
			Community action groups		

[3] This survey is adapted from Janice Matsutsuyu, "The Interest Check List," *American Journal of Occupational Therapy*, 13, 4:323–328 (1969).

find particularly enjoyable. Thus, an asterisk (*) is sometimes placed after each activity that the patient actually enjoys.

To determine whether the patient's recreational activities are appropriate and adequate either now or for the future, the therapist asks herself: "Are these activities typical for an individual of the patient's age, sex, and cultural background?" "Do or will these activities provide the type of satisfaction most people receive from recreational activities?" There is much individual variation in the area of recreation. What recreational activities are best and how much time to spend in recreation is different for each individual. The patient and therapist often need to discuss this area in considerable detail.

Intimacy. Intimacy is that area of human experience that involves a close, sustained relationship with other individuals. Friendships, love relationships, and nurturing the growth of a child are common examples of intimacy. As mentioned earlier, the development of intimacy appears to take place in stages. The skills learned at each stage are not lost but become part of the individual's repertoire. This is true for all stages except a chum relationship. The behavior exhibited at this time is usually not repeated after this stage of development has been completed. The therapist usually has little opportunity to observe intimacy directly. Thus, a structured interview is used to discuss this area with the patient. When possible, however, the therapist directly observes a parent with his children. This can be done in the patient's home, during family visiting time at the treatment facility, or by special appointment with the children.

The behavior, ideas, emotions, and values outlined below indicate that an individual has the ability to engage in the various intimate relationships.

Casual friendship: States that he has friends whom he sees regularly, expresses a liking for these friends, and experiences pleasure in being with them; enjoys doing things with his friends as well as just sitting and talking.

Chum relationship: Currently has or had in the past one or two friends with whom he spent considerable time almost every day; if he was unable to be with the friend, he called him for lengthy conversations on the telephone. The individual trusted his friend implicitly and shared very personal information with him. The individual experienced extreme jealousy when he thought his friend was giving too much time or attention to someone else.

Love relationship: The person sees a few other individuals as being particularly important to him, although he may not use the word love to explain the relationship. He talks very much as if he loved these people. He accepts their limitations as well as their assets and is willing to make sacrifices for them. He turns to these people for help with personal problems; the individual feels very close to these friends but does not feel a loss of personal autonomy. There is no jealous possessiveness, and he accepts the fact that these friends may have love relationships with other people.

Nurturing relationship: Experiences great pleasure in taking care of others and helping them to grow. Satisfies the needs of others without expecting reciprocal satisfaction; devotes considerable time and energy to the relationship. Gives unconditional love. Respects the right of the person to be a unique individual; is able to allow the other individual to move out of the nurturing relationship when he is ready to do so.

The Private Self

The private self refers to the cognitive system, emotions, needs, and values. These facets of man are so intertwined with one another, and so closely related to behavior, that isolated evaluation of each area is not recommended. During all of the evaluative procedures previously mentioned, the therapist tries to get a feel for what the patient knows about the world around him and his ideas about himself and other people. She attempts to determine whether the patient is aware of his needs and how he goes about meeting his needs. The therapist tries to discover what emotions the patient is experiencing and how well he is able to express his emotions. Finally, the therapist makes an effort to find out something about the patient's system of values. When a patient has some verbal skill and self-awareness, the therapist is able to be more direct in questioning him about facets of his private self. For example, after participation in a group-interaction skill evaluation group, the therapist might ask the patient to describe his behavior and other group members' responses to him. She might ask him what he thought of other group members, what feelings he experienced while participating in the group, whether he felt that any of his needs were satisfied by other group members, and what was good and bad about the group.

Another method of evaluating facets of the private self is the use of an Activity Configuration [4] like that shown below. This tool can be used to assess a patient's ideas, feelings, need satisfaction, and values relative to his typical weekly activities. In using this tool, the patient and therapist complete Part I of the Activity Configuration together. This involves a

---

[4] This Activity Configuration was adapted from an evaluative tool designed by Sandra Watanaba. Her tool in turn was adapted from a form and interview process developed by Richard Spahn of the Austin-Riggs Foundation, Stockbridge, Massachusetts, 1968.

Activity Configuration

Part I

Time	Mon.	Tues.	Wed.	Thurs.	Fri.	Sat.	Sun.
6–7							
7–8							
8–9							
9–10							
10–11							
11–12							
12–1							
1–2							
2–3							
3–4							
4–5							
5–6							
6–7							
7–8							
8–9							
9–10							
10–11							

Part II

A. What needs does the activity satisfy? What needs are not satisfied during this activity or not satisfied because of engaging in the activity?
B. I have to do this activity. I want to do this activity. Or both?
C. I want to do this activity and I think this is good. I want to do this activity and I think this is not good. Others make me do this and I am glad they do. Or others make me do this and I wish they did not.
D. I do this activity very well. I do this activity well enough. Or I do not do this well enough.
E. I feel joy, liking, love, fear or anxiety, dislike, hatred, anger, depression, guilt, or some other emotion while engaging in this activity. Before and after engaging in this activity, I feel _____ and _____.

detailed listing of all activities that are part of a usual week. Then, using Part II as a guide, the therapist and patient discuss each activity mentioned. They attempt to discover what the patient thinks about each activity, the needs the activity satisfies, what feelings are aroused when participating in the activity, and what value is placed on the activity.

Initial evaluation of facets of the private self is always highly tentative. The therapist is often able to attain only a general impression of the patient's assets and limitations. During the treatment process itself, the therapist and patient will, if the subject is given adequate attention, be able to discover much more about the patient's thinking and feeling and how this influences his behavior.

RECORD KEEPING AND REPORTS

The various surveys, the activity configuration, the questionnaire, if one is used, and any other notes the therapist may have made during evaluation are usually placed in the patient's individual file. These are kept in the activities therapy department. A summary of the evaluation findings is also placed in the file, as well as in the patient's general chart or file which is used by all persons who are involved with the patient.

In the summary, usually entitled "Initial Evaluation," the therapist states which of the various areas were assessed. The patient's assets and limitations are outlined. Some evidence is given for the interpretations that have been made. For example, in describing a patient's ability to carry out a task, the therapist states what the task was and why she felt that the patient did or did not do an adequate job. Similarly, if the therapist believes the patient does not have the ability to interact in a parallel group, she describes specific things the patient did that led her to this conclusion. The summary also includes a tentative statement regarding the expected environment.

Summaries of periodic evaluation are also written and placed in the activities therapy department file and the patient's general file. When the initial evaluation is incomplete, information regarding assessment of additional areas is included in the periodic evaluation summaries. The format outlined above is also used for writing periodic evaluative findings. The periodic reports indicate what changes have occurred in the patient's problem areas, whether new goals are to be established, and any changes in the treatment plan. This is discussed in more detail in Chapter 7.

Record keeping and writing reports is often seen as a deadly chore by many therapists. It is time consuming, and it does require a degree of self-discipline. However, in a more positive light, written evaluation summaries help the patient and therapist identify assets that can be utilized by the patient and remind them of problem areas that need to be altered, if possible. Keeping all this informtion in mind for many patients is very difficult. Much can be overlooked if it is not written down.

SUGGESTED READING

Fidler, G., and Fidler, J. *Occupational Therapy: A Communication Process in Psychiatry.* New York: Macmillan Company, 1963.

Matsutsuyu, Janice. "The Interest Check List," *American Journal of Occupational Therapy,* 13, 4: 323–328 (1969).

Tyler, Leona. *Tests and Measurements.* Englewood Cliffs, N.J.: Prentice-Hall, 1971.

CHAPTER 7

THE TREATMENT PROCESS

Treatment is a planned collaborative interaction between the therapist, the patient, and the nonhuman environment directed toward the development of skills for community living. This brief chapter discusses the treatment process in general. The following chapters focus more specifically on development of basic skills and facets of the public and private self. Treatment involves the following sequence of events: (1) setting immediate and long-term goals; (2) writing a treatment plan; (3) implementing the treatment plan; (4) periodic evaluation; (5) alteration of goals and the treatment process; and (6) decision making regarding the patient's readiness for discontinuation of treatment.

A *goal* is a definite end toward which treatment is directed. The immediate goal is the area of difficulty with which the patient and therapist decide to deal at a given time in treatment. The long-term goals are to eliminate or minimize all areas of difficulty. They are set in relationship to the patient's expected environment. The patient and therapist together decide what the goals of treatment will be. This is done by reviewing the information gained in the initial evaluation. Areas of difficulty are identified and priorities are set. Goals are written and become part of the patient's file. These goals, of course, may change as the patient and therapist identify additional problem areas or decide that a different expected future environment would be more suitable for the patient. In writing down the goals, the patient and therapist are essentially entering into an agreement. This is a contract established between the therapist and the patient.

There are times when the therapist and the patient do not entirely agree about what should and should not be a goal of treatment. These areas of disagreement are left open for further discussion at a later time. Treatment is initially directed toward a goal for which there is mutual agreement.

Occasionally a patient is just not able to enter into discussion regarding goals. The therapist then sets at least an immediate goal and begins treatment. The patient is told the immediate goal even if he does not seem able to understand it. Goal setting is discussed with the patient when he appears ready for such a discussion.

Ideally, goals are stated concretely, in terms of what the patient is going to be able to do or what he is not going to do any longer. A poor example of a goal is "to develop better work habits." A better example is "to arrive at a community job placement on time," or "to do assigned work tasks without arguing about the assignment." Concrete statements of goals are preferred because the patient and the therapist are more easily able to determine whether or not the goal has been attained.

The *treatment plan* is a written statement of what the patient and the therapist intend to do to attain the goals that have been set. When a treatment center is structured so that there are previously established groups designed to help patients with various problem areas, the treatment plan states in which groups the patient will participate. For example, if the patient has difficulty using his leisure time in a need-satisfying manner, he may be placed in an on-going group that is actively exploring recreational facilities in the community. Or a patient who appears to misperceive common events may be encouraged to join a cooking group in which the leader and participants devote considerable time to talking about what is going on in the immediate situation.

When the patient's areas of difficulty are such that they require treatment in a one-to-one situation, the treatment plan outlines what the patient and therapist will do. Larry, for example, appeared to be unable to do even very simple tasks. He could not make his bed, complete a link belt, or wash dishes. The treatment plan listed various tasks sequentially from fairly easy to more difficult that Larry would learn how to do. These were tasks Larry had mentioned he would like to be able to do. Further, the plan said that the therapist would demonstrate each task and help Larry do each task a few times. Larry was to receive a token every time he participated for three minutes in a way that was likely to lead to task accomplishment. The number of tokens he received during each learning session determined how many records he was allowed to listen to in the evening.

To illustrate further, Enid was overwhelmed by the job of taking care of three young children and an apartment in a slum neighborhood. The treatment plan stated that the therapist would work with Enid in her home to establish task priorities and a weekly schedule. Enid would also be helped to simplify household chores and, if she requested, be given advice about disciplining and playing with her children.

The treatment plan is discussed with the patient. He is helped to see the relationship between the goals which he helped to set and what he and the therapist will be doing to reach these goals. The various groups in which he will be participating are described, and his role in each group is outlined. The patient may suggest changes in the treatment plan, and these changes are made if at all possible. At the end of this discussion regarding treatment, the patient is sometimes given a weekly schedule telling him the day, time, and place of meetings of groups in which he will be participating, meetings he is required to attend, and individual treatment sessions. A weekly schedule is particularly useful if the treatment facility is large or if the patient seems to be confused or has difficulty remembering things. For many patients, a written weekly schedule provides a sense of security; they know what to expect.

The treatment plan is *implemented* as soon as possible. The plan is usually followed as it was initially stated until the first periodic evaluation. However, if the patient is not participating in the plan—not attending assigned groups, for example, or being physically present but not actively engaging in activities—the therapist investigates the situation. An attempt is made to identify the reasons for nonparticipation. The patient's comments about his reasons for not participating are listened to with great care. Disregard of this information frequently interferes with the treatment process. If necessary, the treatment plan is changed to be more compatible with the patient's desires. Often, however, the patient simply needs additional encouragement. This is particularly true at the beginning of the treatment process, when the patient is entering a completely new situation and is being asked to learn things that are very difficult for him to do.

Periodic evaluation takes place at least once a month, if not more frequently. It is a rather formal procedure, and a definite time is set aside for the evaluation. Ideally, the patient and all of the people who are involved in his treatment are present. All problem areas are reassessed to determine what, if any, changes have taken place. When the immediate goals of treatment have been reached, more advanced goals are set. A new plan is written and treatment continues. That is the ideal sequence of events. However, it is sometimes discovered that the patient really has not changed since the initial evaluation or last periodic evaluation. It also may appear that the patient has more problem areas than those originally identified.

If treatment is not progressing in the anticipated manner, the patient and therapist need to look at: (1) the type and amount of medication the patient is receiving; (2) the immediate goal(s); (3) the treatment situation(s); and (4) elements outside the treatment situation. It is possible that the patient might receive more benefit from another kind of medication. On the other hand, the patient may be taking too much or not enough medication. The responsible physician is consulted. The immediate goal for treatment may have been set too high. That is, the goal may have been too advanced for the patient to reach at the present time. When this is the case, simpler or more basic goals are set, a new plan is written, and treatment continues. At other times, it may be found that the immediate goal is not truly compatible with the patient's wishes. He may have thought that he wanted to reach the stated goal, but he may not really want to do so. Another goal is then selected for the present. To discover factors that are interfering with treatment, it is often helpful to compare the treatment situation to the principles of the teaching-learning process outlined in Chapter 3. Perhaps crucial principles are not being used or one principle needs to be emphasized more than it has been. Similarly, one might look at the factors that interfere with group functioning outlined in Chapter 4. For example, are there group norms that inhibit change, or is the communication process faulty? When factors in the treatment situation are found to be interfering with learning, the therapist and patient attempt to make the necessary changes.

Some elements outside the treatment situation that may interfere with treatment are as follows:

1. There may be divergent ideas about treatment. This may occur, for example, when some of the staff believe that the use of therapeutic drugs is the only type of treatment that is effective, or that only in-depth psychotherapy will alter behavior. When some staff members hold either of these beliefs, they tend to view activities therapy as "keeping the patients occupied." This attitude may be communicated to the patients. Thus, the patients may experience conflict, hesitating to devote time and energy to the activities therapy program.

2. The atmosphere of the treatment facility or the current life situation

of the patient may not be conducive to treatment. Decisions about a patient's privilege or discharge date may be made in a highly arbitrary manner, for example, or there may be an excessive number of rules and regulations. Patients cannot participate in treatment if their basic human needs are not being met or if they are preoccupied with personal crises. An example of the latter would be concern about a severely ill parent or imminent loss of usual income.

3. People important to the patient may indicate in some way that they do not wish the patient to change. A patient's wife, for example, may become frightened when her dependent and possessive husband begins to assert himself. She does not know how to cope with this new behavior and indicates to the patient that she is more comfortable with his former behavior.

When the patient and therapist find any of these factors interfering with the treatment process, they work together to bring about the necessary changes. Identification of these factors alone may be sufficient to allow treatment to continue. However, these disruptive factors cannot always be altered, or at least not at the present time. It may be necessary for treatment to be discontinued. Sometimes we just cannot treat a patient. This is an unhappy fact of life a therapist must somehow accept.

If the initial evaluation was incomplete, other facets of the patient's abilities may be investigated at the time of a periodic evaluation. The therapist, for example, might feel that a patient is now ready to examine his ability to work or to explore the ways in which he has used his leisure time. A periodic evaluation also offers an opportunity to reassess the patient's expected environment. Should it be the same as the one identified at the time of the initial evaluation or the last periodic evaluation? The patient or therapist may feel that the previously agreed-upon expected environment will not give sufficient support to the patient. Or, the proposed expected environment may be too sheltered; the patient might be more comfortable in a living situation that allows for more independence and decision making. Finally, the patient's interests and values may have changed. For example, Rosemary may now feel that she does not want to return to college, or George may have decided that he will try a senior citizens' residence. When the expected environment is to be different from the one originally planned, the patient's assets and limitations must be reassessed relative to the new expected environment. Does the patient need less, more, or different skills for this new environment?

It may be necessary to set different long-term treatment goals.

The final phase of the treatment process is to assess whether the patient is ready to discontinue treatment. This is essentially an on-going process which is discussed at each periodic evaluation. The major question therapist and patient ask is, "Can the patient function in his expected environment?" Leaving a treatment facility can be an anxiety-provoking event. Thus, the experience is frequently graduated to allow the patient to spend increasing amounts of time in the community. He is encouraged to participate in all aspects of the life situation to which he will return. A patient often needs additional support at this time. He may become concerned about his ability to function and return temporarily to old patterns of behavior. The therapist helps the patient at this time by honest reassurance and continual feedback about the patient's ability to function.

SUGGESTED READING

Brammer, L., and Shostrom, E. *Therapeutic Psychology.* Englewood Cliffs, N.J.: Prentice-Hall, 1968.

Combs, A., Avila, D., and Purkey, W. *Helping Relationships.* Boston: Allyn & Bacon, 1971.

Grosser, C., Henery, W., and Kelly, J. *Nonprofessionals in the Human Services.* San Francisco: Jossey-Boss, 1969.

Mager, Robert. *Preparing Instructional Objectives.* Palo Alto, Calif.: Fearon Publishers, 1962.

Willard, H., and Spackman, C. *Occupational Therapy* (4th ed.). Philadelphia: J. B. Lippincott Co., 1971.

CHAPTER 8

DEVELOPMENT OF BASIC SKILLS

The learning of simple task skills and the lower-level group-interaction skills is usually the first goal of treatment if a patient lacks these abilities. Priority is often given to simple task skills. When a patient lacks simple task skills, he is usually unable to participate in a parallel group. So much energy and attention must be focused on the task that the patient tends to ignore the other people in the group.

In this chapter and the two chapters that follow, treatment is usually described as taking place in specially designed learning situations. And this is, in truth, where much of patient learning occurs. However, the casual, everyday interactions of patients and staff members are also sometimes used for learning. Situations may arise while doing morning chores, over a leisurely lunch, or during a late evening chat that can be used to enhance development. For example, while preparing to go for a walk, Claude was gently reminded that perhaps he should put on shoes rather than wear slippers. At dinner one evening, Delia complained at length about her inadequacies in dealing with a hospital job. Finally the therapist, in a joking manner, said, "All right, you have told us all the things you can't do, now why don't you give us a list of what you can do." Spontaneous learning situations provide an opportunity for growth and development in many areas. The therapist takes advantage of these situations whenever possible. However, there is a limit. The patient should not be nudged every moment of the day. That is too much for anyone. For example, in one day treatment center, patients and staff members solved this problem by decreeing that the usual after-lunch volleyball game was "off limits." It was not to be used for learning; it was for relaxation and fun.

TASK SKILLS

There seem to be two kinds of difficulties with regard to task skills. There are patients who appear unable to do even the most simple task. They usually show little interest in doing anything. Other patients engage in activities, but are deficient in some aspect of the doing process: They work too fast, give up when they come to a snag, or do a sloppy job. However, regardless of the type of difficulty, the three major points to remember are the following:

1. Try to find some activity that interests the patient. Try anything —even things that you do not especially like to do or that you find dull and boring.
2. Start where the patient is and move slowly from there.
3. Provide considerable reinforcement for even very small changes.

Patients who have difficulty doing simple tasks need support and encouragement. Frequently, the therapist must spend considerable time establishing a relationship of basic trust between herself and the patient. The patient may be suspicious of attention and feel that other people do not understand how difficult it is for him to do anything that requires overt, self-initiated action. In order to build trust, the therapist may initially spend only a few moments with the patient, being silent if the patient seems to prefer that level of interaction. Later, she may talk quietly about small events on the ward, such as what was for lunch and/or a ward attendant's new moustache. Sometimes, it is helpful to bring something the patient seems to like—a piece of candy, a cigarette, or a stick of gum. Later, in this tenuous relationship, the therapist may give her usual small gift only after the patient looks at her or says hello. Slowly and carefully, the therapist build the relationship. Minimal demands are made. The first thing the patient and therapist might do besides simply being with each other is to take a walk or go to the canteen for coffee. Introduction of a task may mean simply tossing a ball back and forth or playing one-finger duets on the piano. The task is mutually shared. Later, the therapist introduces tasks in which the patient independently does one part while the therapist does another part. For example, the patient picks out the right color tile for a checkered tile ashtray while the therapist glues the tile into the form, or the patient dips the ginger cookie balls into the sugar after the therapist has formed the dough into balls. Finally, the patient is encouraged to do simple tasks alone, such as molding a bowl out of clay or lacing up a precut leather coin case . . . and so forth, through a small step by small step process.

Some patients who have difficulty with even simple tasks function at a higher interpersonal level. They are able to establish a trust relationship much more quickly, but only if no demands are made for task performance. They have a fair degree of verbal skill. Often, in fact, they are much better at talking than at doing. The problem with these patients seems to be that doing any task with an end result that can be judged (i.e., are the dishes clean, did the ball get into the basket, etc.) is frightening. The patient, often unbeknown to himself, has established relationships such as, "If I do something well, people will expect me to do everything well," or, "Any negative judgment about anything I do means I am totally and absolutely no good." These essentially false cognitive relationships need to be altered. But this is the kind of patient who may be helped to become aware of and talk about how he sees himself and the world, with no effort toward action. He discusses his difficulties freely, thinking, somehow, that they will magically disappear if he simply talks about them. What this type of patient seems to need is a lot less talking and a lot more doing. But slowly. There needs to be graduated movement into anything that might be judged. For example, spontaneous free movement to music or "playing" with finger painting might be the beginning. This is safe: No one can say a free movement is good or bad. And everyone knows finger painting is for children; it is easy to throw away, no one cares, it is not like a real painting. The therapist waits. Given time, the patient is more than likely to say, "That felt good for that part of the music, I'll try it again," or "I like that finger painting, let's keep it." The patient is beginning to make his own judgments. The therapist works from there, moving slowly from tasks that require self-judgment to tasks that can be judged by some measurable standard. A person's ideas about relationships are often changed only when he experiences a different, more accurate relationship.

The other kind of patients mentioned were those who have difficulty with one or more aspects of doing a task. Appropriate activities for correcting a problem area will depend on what the patient needs to learn. The following suggestions may be useful.

Rate of Performance

Faulty rate of performance means that a person works too fast or too slowly in performing a task. Telling a patient to work more quickly or slowly may help, but this often begins to sound like nagging. If a patient works too slowly, a time limit of three minutes may be set in the initial stages of treatment. The patient is asked to do a part of a task that takes approximately three minutes to do when it is done at a normal rate. If he finishes the assigned task in the specified time, he is given some sort of reinforcement. If he goes not finish the task, a shorter time period is set. The patient is allowed to rest for a few minutes and is then asked to work another three minutes, and so on until the task is finished. Each day the time periods are increased in length. The task should be short-term; the patient should be able to finish it in one treatment session. This helps the patient acquire a sense of accomplishment. The patient is never allowed to work on the task at his usual slow rate during the treatment period. Doing so may reinforce his slowness. Simple tasks are usually best at the first stage of treatment so the patient does not get slowed down by having to figure out what to do.

When a patient works too quickly, he usually has a considerable amount of excess energy. He may find it more comfortable to do tasks that require vigorous gross movements, such as playing touch football or moving furniture. This may provide an excellent source of reinforcement. The patient is initially asked to do a task at a normal rate for a short period of time and then allowed to engage in a task that requires vigorous gross movement. The time period for doing a task at a normal rate prior to reinforcement is increased as treatment continues. The task is kept simple in the initial phase of treatment so that the patient is confronted with as few problems as possible.

Appropriate Use of Tools and Materials

There seem to be two problems related to difficulty in using tools and materials in an appropriate manner. In some cases the patient simply does not know how to use many tools and materials. In other cases the patient knows how to use tools and materials but does not take the time or effort to use them in an appropriate manner. The therapist and patient have to determine which problem the patient is having or whether the problem is a combination of not knowing and not taking enough time.

When the patient does not know how to use tools and materials, he is helped to learn. Learning is usually achieved within the context of an activity rather than through repetition with no purpose other than learning to use a tool or material. For example, a therapist demonstrates how to use a ruler. She may ask the patient to draw a few lines of specified length, but there is no long period of practice. Rather, the therapist has the patient start to make a cardboard pattern for a billfold he wants to make. Only one or two tools or materials that the patient does not know how to use should be introduced in each new activity. The other aspects of the task should be familiar to the patient. For example, if a patient knows absolutely nothing about cooking, learning starts with opening a can of soup, adding the necessary water, heating the soup, and eating it. Learning does not begin with making a cake from scratch.

Appropriate use of tools and materials does not mean that there is one right way to do everything. Rather, there are limits. There are, for example, several ways to clean a paint brush, but it must be cleaned if it is going to be used again. A pan used to cook oatmeal is much easier to clean if it is soaked in cold water than a pan that is not soaked. It is nearly impossible to press a rayon blouse when the iron is set for wool. A patient who does not take the time and effort to use tools and materials in an appropriate manner tends to do tasks in such a way that he eventually makes twice as much work either for himself or for someone else. He may damage the tools and materials or handle them in such a way that he is likely to injure himself or others. In helping a patient to use tools and materials in an appropriate manner, the therapist stops the patient each time he does something that is, for example, wasteful or unsafe. She reminds the patient of the "right" way and insists that he do it in the right way. Positive reinforcement is given after the correction has been made. Positive reinforcement and feedback are also given while the patient is doing a task in an acceptable manner. If the therapist pays attention to the patient only when he is doing something wrong, the patient may get in the habit of making mistakes just to receive attention.

Willingness to Engage in Doing Tasks

Patients who show little willingness to engage in tasks have usually experienced little need satisfaction from task-oriented behavior. They prefer to do nothing, or they talk a lot but never seem to get anything done. The goal of treatment in this area is to help a patient realize that doing tasks can be need satisfying. The teaching situation is designed so that the patient experiences need gratification from either the process of doing a task or the end result. Thus, it is important to know what the patient's specific needs are. What does the patient want right now? It is often useful to get a commitment from the patient to do something, a simple thing, anything. It does not really matter what the patient decides to do. The point is that he do some task. The therapist continues to request that the patient make commitments, slowly graduating the requests so that they involve an increasing amount of task-oriented behavior. The need to ask for a formal commitment will hopefully decrease as the patient realizes that task-oriented behavior leads to need satisfaction.

Sustained Interest in a Task

Patients who have difficulty sustaining interest in a task often have a short attention span. They may wander away from the task, begin another task, go to look out the window, daydream, or get involved in a conversation. They may return to the task momentarily, then wander away again. Other patients remain interested in a task for a while, then lose all interest. They want to start another task. Their problem is that they never finish anything. Every undertaking results in an unfinished project.

To help a patient increase his attention span, the therapist and patient may decide how long the patient will work without interruption. This may be for only two or three minutes at the beginning of treatment. Just being able to work for a predetermined period of time may be sufficient reinforcement, or the therapist may have to provide reinforcement. The length of work periods is slowly increased at a rate that is comfortable for the patient. Another method the therapist may use is to pay no attention to the patient when he is not working at whatever he is supposed to be doing. The therapist gives the patient attention and approval only when the patient is engaged in task-oriented behavior.

The therapist can help patients who never seem to be able to finish a task by insisting that they finish each task they start. Sometimes patients do not complete projects because they select ones that take a very long time to complete or ones that are too complex or too repetitive for them. Thus, in the beginning of treatment, the patient is helped to choose a task that is relatively short-term, fairly easy to do, and nonrepetitive. Once a task is chosen, the patient is not permitted to select another task until he has finished the first task. At first, the patient may need help in finishing a task; if so, he is given assistance. However, it is made clear that receiving assistance is only temporary. The patient will, at some point, be expected to finish tasks by himself. As treatment progresses, the patient is encouraged to select tasks that take an increasingly longer time to complete and that are increasingly more complex.

Ability to Follow Demonstrated, Oral, and Written Instructions

Patients who have difficulty following instructions may not be able to follow one type of instruction. For example, a patient may need to be *shown* how to do a task; he does not understand if someone only tells him how to do it. Other patients can follow one-step instructions, but they are not able to follow a list of instructions. The first type of patient may be helped by telling him how to do a task and showing him how to do it at the same time. Slowly the therapist decreases the demonstrated part of the instructions, eventually giving only verbal directions. When the patient is only able to follow one-step instructions, that is where treatment starts. The therapist slowly increases the number of steps, one by one.

Some patients do not bother to read instructions. Or they read the instructions once and then go ahead with the project, never returning to the instructions to check whether they are doing the project correctly. Steps may be forgotten or done out of sequence. Patients need to be reminded to read instructions and to compare what they are doing with the instructions periodically. Other patients repeatedly ask for verbal instructions to be given again. This is often more a way of getting attention than of actually forgetting what was said. If this is the case, it may be useful for the therapist or someone else to stay with the patient after he has been given the instructions. Time spent with the patient is slowly decreased until he is able to work alone for a period of time. It is also important that the patient's need for attention be satisfied in many different interactions in the treatment center.

Acceptable Level of Neatness

Acceptable level of neatness refers to both the neatness of the end product and to whether a person cleans up after he has finished a task. Patients who have difficulty creating a neat end product can be helped initially by involving them in tasks that require little neatness, for example, painting a bookcase that is standing on a lot of newspaper as opposed to painting the area around a window. The patient is slowly introduced to tasks that require increasing neatness. The patient is encouraged to work neatly and is given adequate instructions about how to do the task in a neat manner. When a sloppy end product can be changed to make it look neater, the patient is urged to make these changes. When a patient does not seem to have any idea about what is or is not neatly done, the therapist sets standards for him. She then gives the patient feedback about whether or not he has met the standards.

It is rather generally accepted that a person can be as sloppy as he wants to while doing a task if he cleans up when he is finished. Besides stating this norm clearly, the therapist may find it useful to use shaping. The therapist initially helps a patient to pick up and reinforces any attempts the patient makes at cleaning up. Approximations of the desired behavior are reinforced. The therapist slowly decreases her participation in cleaning up as the patient is more able to take on responsibility. The therapist also may help patients learn to do tasks in such a way that cleaning up is easier, for example, to put the spoon used to stir the spaghetti sauce on a plate rather than several different places on the counter, or to put newspapers on the table before starting a project that requires the use of glue. Patients are encouraged to think about cleaning up before they start a task to see if there are ways of doing the task that will make cleanup less of a chore.

Appropriate Attention to Detail

Appropriate attention to detail means knowing the difference between straightening up a room and giving a room a thorough cleaning. Patients who have difficulty in this area tend to be compulsive. Every detail is important. They will spend hours trying to make something perfect. These patients need to be encouraged to try not to be so concerned with detail, to be a little less neat, to leave something undone for the time being. The patient is likely to need a considerable amount of reinforcement and reassurance that nothing horrible is going to happen if he does not do something perfectly.

Solves Problems That Arise in Performing a Task

Patients who have difficulty in problem solving tend to give up on a task if they encounter any problems, or they immediately ask for help.

They make no attempt to figure out how to solve the problem. The learning situation, therefore, is designed so that the patient moves slowly from tasks that usually present very few problems to tasks that require a fair amount of problem solving. Activities are graduated. For example, the patient might start by cutting and sewing a felt vest, move on to making a two-piece cotton shift with no fastening, to a long skirt with a zipper, to a shirt with a collar and buttons.

In addition to graduating tasks, the therapist encourages the patient to reread the instructions or to go to another book for instructions. When the patient is afraid to try something new on the item he is making, he is urged to try it out first on something else. Using the example above, it might be suggested to the patient that he make a buttonhole on a scrap of cloth before he tries to make one in his shirt. Patients are helped to study a problem, to look closely at what is involved, to identify specifically what the problem is, to think of various courses of action to take, and to determine the consequence of various ways of solving a problem. When the therapist must solve a problem for a patient, she tries to explain how and why she arrived at a particular solution.

Organizes Task in a Logical Manner

Organization of tasks refers to such things as, for example, being sure you have all the ingredients before starting to make fudge, getting all the equipment and materials together before sitting down to make a poster, or washing the bathroom sink before washing the tile floor. Patients who have difficulty in this area must be helped to think about a task before they begin. They are encouraged to identify and locate all the items they will need for task completion and to consider what should be done first, second, and so forth.

In the above discussion, the teaching of each aspect of task skills was discussed separately. However, patients who have difficulty in the area of task skills often have trouble with several aspects of the skill. For example, they may not be able to sustain interest in a task or to give appropriate attention to detail. In designing a learning situation, the therapist may want to help a patient with all his deficits in the area of task skills at the same time or deal with only one area at a time. The decision will depend on whether the areas for learning are compatible. For example, the therapist would probably not be concerned about task neatness when she was trying to get a patient to engage in a task, any task. However, it would be fairly easy to teach the appropriate use of tools and materials and problem solving at the same time.

In the above discussion, there was little mention of how changing a person's thinking, feelings, and values will lead to change in the area of task skills. This is discussed in some detail in Chapter 10. For now, it suffices to say that in activities therapy it is not assumed that a change in thinking, feelings, and values automatically leads to a change in behavior. For example, Sylvia realizes that she has used her scatterbrain, inept image as a way of getting acceptance and decides that she no longer wants to be this way. This does not mean that Sylvia will immediately be able to organize tasks in a logical manner and solve problems that arise in performing a task. Conversely, it is not assumed that a change in behavior automatically leads to a change in thinking, feelings, or values. For example, helping Jacob learn how to carry a task through to the end may do little to influence his belief that completing a task means you are one step closer to death. Activities therapy assumes a reciprocal relationship between the private self and the other two facets of man—basic skills and the public self.

GROUP-INTERACTION SKILLS

Ideally, patients are helped to learn group-interaction skills in groups specially designed to teach one level of group-interaction skill and nothing else. Patients are placed in a group that is functioning at one level above the level of group-interaction skill the patient appears to have reached at the time of initial evaluation. For example, if the patient has the ability to interact in a parallel group, he is placed in a group at the project level. The group as a whole may continue to learn the remaining group-interaction skills together, but only if all patients in a group learn at about the same rate. Or a patient, after mastering the subskill taught in his present group, may move into another group which is functioning at the next level. The only treatment facility organization that seems to allow for this way of teaching group-interactions skill is that in which the activities therapy department is centralized, as in a large unit of a general hospital.

In the other types of treatment facility organizations, a patient is placed in a group that may or may not be functioning at his level of group-interaction skill. Groups such as the daily living group and the small morning group described in Chapter 5 are usually approximately at the egocentric-cooperative group level. This is fine for the initial learning of the patient who has the ability to participate in a project group, but it raises some difficulty for the learning of patients who are at a different level. Beginning and more advanced skills are either taught in this middle-range group, in a pure group (i.e., groups specially designed to teach one level of group-interaction skill) in the treatment center, or in a group outside the treatment facility.

Regardless of what level of group-interaction skill the therapist is at-tempting to develop, she designs the learning situation so that the patient (1) is both aware of and helped to engage in appropriate behavior and (2) receives reinforcement of, or feedback about, his behavior or both. The therapist tells a patient what behavior is expected of him before he enters a group and periodically reminds group members of what is and is not appropriate behavior in the group. Before a patient can receive reinforce-ment for a desired behavior, the behavior must occur. The therapist may simply wait for an approximation of a desirable behavior and then rein-force that behavior selectively. This is the process of shaping. But just waiting for an approximation of desirable behavior can take a long time. There are several other methods a therapist may use. One is to encourage the patient to imitate another group member who is functioning fairly well in the group. Or the therapist may suggest to a patient that he try to act in a particular way, giving him ideas about what he might say and do. A way of acting that is ineffective or inappropriate for the group may be pointed out to the patient. The patient is encouraged to interact in a different manner, without any specific suggestions being given. Trial-and-error learning is encouraged, with the patient receiving feedback about the appropriateness of his experimental behavior. Or the group may pause periodically in their activity to examine what behavior has been useful to the group and the individual and what behavior has been harmful or of minimal use to the group or the individual. This process both reinforces the learning of appropriate behavior and gives group members clues as to the kinds of behavior they might try. A discussion of this kind is kept as nonpersonal as possible. Group members are not singled out and told they did something right or wrong. Although using immediate examples of what occurred in the group, the discussion is oriented to talking about what kind of behavior is useful in this type of group and what behavior is not useful. Discussion is more academic than personal.

Finally, the group may discontinue its current activity and experiment with various ways of acting through role-playing exercises. Role playing may center around an incident that has just occurred within the group. For example, Jerome wanted to ask Beth a question and interrupted her while she was talking to another group member. Beth, very abruptly, told Jerome to get lost. Various group members took both Jerome's and Beth's parts, role playing both ways of getting attention so you can ask a question and ways of responding to interruptions without hurting the other person's feelings. On the other hand, a role-playing exercise may focus on a general problem within the group. For example, the group may have decided that one of its difficulties is that group members are afraid to express definite opinions about anything. Role playing then may be an attempt to study ways of stating ideas directly. The role playing is designed to allow group members to experiment both with expressing an opinion and with how to respond to the expression of a personal opinion.

As mentioned in Chapter 3, reinforcement and feedback are very important in the teaching-learning process. The therapist may have to take responsibility for this aspect of learning, but ideally she enlists the help of all group members. This is done by assisting group members not only to understand what is appropriate behavior for a particular group, but also assisting them to learn to give and withhold reinforcement and to provide feedback. If it seems appropriate, a new group may spend their first few meetings learning about reinforcement and feedback. Review of this learning may need to take place when new patients come into the group, or when it is evident that some group members are having difficulty providing reinforcement and feedback.

The following paragraphs suggest ways of helping a patient learn each of the group-interaction skills.

Ability to Participate in a Parallel Group

Some patients are not ready to begin learning how to participate in a parallel group. They are either so suspicious or so unaware of other people that they have little interest in interacting in a group. When the organization of the treatment center does not demand that a patient be placed into a group, it is usually better for patients who are not ready to start learning group-interaction skills to be treated individually. Treatment would be devoted to development of basic trust between patient and therapist and to the learning of simple task skills if necessary. When a patient who is not ready to learn group-interaction skills must be placed in a middle-range group as soon as he comes to the treatment center, few demands for participation are made initially. The patient is welcomed by group members and is given attention and support. He may be excused from participating in the group task or be given considerable assistance by the therapist. The therapist is usually the person to provide assistance, because she is able to give unconditional love. Unconditional love is a prerequisite for developing basic trust. Only after a patient really trusts another person is he ready to begin learning to participate in a parallel group. Some patients are able to give unconditional love. If they so desire, they may be the person with whom the patient is encouraged to develop a basic trust relationship.

When a patient is ready to begin learning how to participate in a parallel group and is to learn this subskill in a pure group, he is prepared for the new experience. The therapist tells the patient what the new group will be like, what kinds of activities the group members do, and what will be expected of him by the group. He is introduced to the therapist who is responsible for the group if he does not know this person already. The therapist is definitely the leader of a parallel group, because patients in the group are able to play very few group-membership roles. Group members' needs for safety, love and acceptance, and esteem are met by the therapist. The therapist reinforces any behavior appropriate for a parallel group—looking at a group member or his task, making eye contact, smiling and laughing appropriately, going to sit next to someone, asking a question, answering a question, making casual conversation, and so forth. The process of shaping is often used. Usually, the therapist ignores inappropriate behavior. However, when the behavior is actually disruptive to the group, the therapist asks the patient either to stop whatever he is doing or to leave the room. Patients who continually disrupt a parallel group are probably not yet ready to learn this skill.

The therapist helps patients to select individual activities and gives them assistance in carrying out the activity. The activities suggested to each patient are kept well within his ability. When a task is fairly easy for a patient to do, it will not require his full attention. Thus, the patient is more likely to interact with other group members. Activities suggested to patients are ones that increase the possibilities of interaction. Activities that must be done in a special area or at an individual table are discouraged, as are activities that take up a large area. For example, a copper enamel kiln is often kept in a special area. Looms are frequently set on individual tables. Because of the nature of the activity, the patient tends to work alone, having little contact with other patients. When a patient is doing an activity that requires a large work area, other patients tend to move away from the table or not join the patient. Therefore, activities such as painting a shoe rack and making a vase using the coil method of construction are not very good activities to suggest. However, if a number of group members want to work with clay, for example, one or two tables may be set aside for their use. In this case, working with clay would be an activity to be encouraged. Two or more patients doing the same type of activity often increases interaction. The patients share something in common; they have something to talk about.

When a patient is to learn to participate in a parallel group in a middle-range group, the therapist and other group members encourage and reinforce behavior that is appropriate for interaction in a parallel group. They are concerned with helping the patient to work at a task in the presence of other group members, to be aware of other group members, and to have some sort of minimal interactions with others. Additional demands for more advanced group-interaction skills are kept to a minimum. When it is impossible for the patient to have an individual task, the person who shares the task with the patient should be aware that the patient has little idea about how to share. The other person will have to take the major responsibility for organizing the task in such a way that the patient can participate. The other person may have to do most of the work. Group members must be aware that a person who does not have the ability to participate in a parallel group often does not know how to ask for or obtain need satisfaction without outside help. Need satisfaction must be provided by group members. Patients in the process of acquiring parallel group skill are unlikely to be active participants in the other learning experiences of a middle-range group, except, perhaps, for the learning of task skills. These patients are usually not yet ready to focus on the development of facets of the private and public self. This is also often true for patients who do not have the ability to participate in a project group.

Ability to Participate in a Project Group

The therapist continues to be a definite leader in a pure project group; she is the major source of need satisfaction for group members. Behavior appropriate for a project group is reinforced by the therapist and other group members if they are able to do so. Examples of behavior that is reinforced are two or more patients doing a task together, cooperation and sharing, mild competition, giving and seeking assistance, and simple interaction beyond the requirements of the task.

The therapist helps group members select short-term tasks that either allow for or require the participation of two or more persons. "Short-term" usually means tasks that require interaction for less than half an hour. This is, of course, an arbitrary period of time. The point is that patients at this level are frequently not able to sustain interaction with the same group of people for a long period of time. For a task that takes longer than half an hour, the therapist usually breaks up the activity so that part of the task is done one day and another part is done the next time the group meets. A patient is often involved in a number of shared tasks in one group session. Group meetings are kept fluid, with a number of small groups participating in a variety of activities. Only occasionally does the group perform an activity that involves the whole group working together at a shared task. The skill required to operate successfully in a group of twelve to fifteen people is usually not available to a person at the project group level.

It is also important that activities be sharable. For example, three or four people making a cake together borders on the ridiculous. Simple team sports and games are good for project groups. Some examples are relay races, volleyball, mixed-doubles badminton, croquet, red rover, pool, card games, and the like. Other activities that might be used are preparing for a short skit, a rhythm band, group singing, making holiday decorations, a shared woodworking project, or preparing a meal.

The goal of a pure project group is to help patients learn how to participate in a shared task. Finishing the task in a given period of time or creating a perfect end product is not emphasized. The therapist gives group members plenty of opportunity to experiment with ways of sharing. Trial-and-error behavior is encouraged. The therapist stresses the idea that if a task does not get done or the results of the task leave something to be desired, there will always be a chance to try again.

When a patient is to learn how to participate in a project group in a middle-range group, the therapist and other patients encourage and reinforce behavior that is appropriate for interacting in a project group. Doing short-term tasks with others is emphasized. Above and beyond the task, the patient is helped to remain aware of other group members, to ask and respond to questions, and to follow along with what the group is doing. However, more complex interpersonal behavior is not required. Group members continue to attempt to identify and meet the patient's needs without asking that the patient be very explicit in stating his needs. If possible, the patient is involved in shared tasks that are not pressured by time or need for perfection.

Ability to Participate in an Egocentric-Cooperative Group

In a pure group designed to teach egocentric-cooperative skills, the therapist takes much less of a leadership role. What the therapist does is finely tuned to what group members are able or almost able to do. The therapist ceases to play a group membership role or takes on a membership role according to the learning needs of the group. The idea is to allow the group to function as independently of the therapist's direction as possible without letting it flounder to the point of disruption. Patients are not given immediate assistance, but neither are they left totally without help.

The therapist and group members reinforce any behavior that leads to successful selection, planning, and carrying out of relatively long-term tasks. The therapist takes primary responsibility for organizing an activity in a project group; in an egocentric-cooperative group, however, group members are helped to take primary responsibility. Initially, group members may need considerable assistance in planning an activity. The therapist may make several suggestions and ask the patients to select an activity from the suggested list, or just two activities may be suggested. Or the group members may be asked to throw out any idea that comes to mind without prejudgment as to whether it is a good or bad suggestion. The group may need information from the therapist about how to arrive at a decision and the different types of decisions. In planning the activity, group members may require help in considering all aspects of the task— what tool and materials will be needed and how to get them, in what order the activity should be carried out, how long it will take, and so forth. While group members are participating in doing the activity, the therapist may need to give encouragement when the going gets rough or interest wanes, guide the group in problem solving, give individual help to one member who is having trouble, and so on. As group members learn to select, plan, and implement a long-term task, the therapist gives increasingly less assistance. Eventually, the therapist serves more as a resource person, relative to the task, than as a group leader.

Almost any activity that allows or requires people to work together is suitable for learning egocentric-cooperative group skills. There are some things to be avoided, however. Repetition of similar types of activities limits the opportunity for group problem solving. Too many activities that involve each group member making something for himself tend to minimize interaction. Spectator-type activities decrease the sense of mutual self-involvement and responsibility. At the beginning of the treatment process, it is often better to do activities that can be completed in one or two meetings of the group. Long, involved projects which take several days are better left until later in the treatment process.

In addition to developing group task skills, the therapist is concerned with helping patients to meet esteem needs through group interaction. Patients are assisted in learning how to state their own need for recognition of achievement, and to identify and meet the esteem needs of other group members. The therapist may act as a model, expressing her own need for recognition and fulfilling the esteem needs of other group members. Reinforcement and feedback relative to esteem needs are provided. The group as a whole might address themselves to such questions as, "How do you indicate that you want someone to give you recognition and praise?" "What does someone look like when they want their esteem needs to be gratified?" or "How do you let someone know he is doing a good job?"

The area of group norms and group members' rights and responsibilities is an important component of egocentric-cooperative group skill. Reinforcement is given for identifying and following group norms, for demanding that one's rights be respected, and for taking responsibility for respecting the rights of others. In parallel and project groups, these behaviors are reinforced by the therapist. But in an egocentric-cooperative group, more conscious attention is given to these matters. The group may take time to talk about the norms of their group, to identify what their group's norms are, to discuss whether and how a norm helps the group to function, or to compare the norms of their group with other groups with which they are familiar. It is helpful if the group has an opportunity consciously to establish a norm. Rights and responsibilities are also discussed, such as, for example, whether Shirley has the right not to attend a meeting of the group for no other reason than that she just does not feel like coming, or whether she has the responsibility of attending all meetings unless she is sick.

Group members are encouraged to accept each individual in the group. They are given help in learning how to show acceptance to fellow group members. However, at this level of group-interaction skill, the therapist continues to meet group members' needs for love and safety. With so much emphasis on the development of group task skills, the patient needs to know he is appreciated for himself regardless of his capacity in the area of doing. Meeting safety needs is important for an egocentric-cooperative learning group. In order to feel free to experiment with group task skills, the group must have a sense that there is someone who will not let them go too far or get into serious trouble. That does not mean the therapist does not ask the group to consider the consequence of what they are doing. It means the group knows the therapist will, if at all possible, identify any harmful consequences they did not take into consideration.

Developing the ability to participate in an egocentric-cooperative group in a middle-range group is fairly simple. A middle-range group functions approximately at an egocentric-cooperative group level. The patient is being asked to participate in a type of group that is only one level above the group skill he already has, so few special precautions have to be taken. The patient is helped to learn how to participate in the life of the group. In terms of the other facets of man the group is designed to develop, the patient may have some difficulty in the areas of intimacy, expressing emotions, and needs. Learning how to participate in a cooperative group contributes to the development of these facets of man. A patient who is just learning how to participate in an egocentric-cooperative group has usually not had the opportunity to be an active member of a cooperative group.

Ability to Participate in a Cooperative Group

In a group designed solely for the development of the ability to partici-pate in a cooperative group, the therapist either takes the role of a "benign leader" or an adviser. The term "benign leader" refers to a role in which the therapist is very much a group participant. She expresses her feelings and ideas with relative freedom and avoids any authoritarian position. In a cooperative group with a benign leader, both therapist and patients take mutual responsibility for reinforcing the behavior to be learned in the group. Some examples of behavior that is reinforced are: from any expression of positive or negative emotions to appropriate expression of emotions, identifying and meeting another person's needs, identifying and expressing one's own needs, and sharing personal feelings and ideas about oneself. Development of a fairly high degree of cohesiveness is important for this type of group. People need a strong sense of trust of and liking for fellow group members if they are going to experiment freely with the expression of very personal aspects of the self. Thus, the therapist helps the group develop a strong sense of identity and specialness.

The best activities for this type of group allow for and encourage expression of feelings. Since the task is secondary to need fulfillment in a cooperative group, activities usually have no significant end product. Examples of useful activities are listening to music, doing individual drawings or paintings, clay modeling, free movement to music or modern dance, or special learning exercises. Special learning exercises are short-term interactions designed to focus on an integrated association of emotions, ideas, values, and needs. One example is to have everyone stand in a circle with one person in the middle. People in the circle first face the center and nonverbally express feelings of love and acceptance for the person in the middle. At a signal from someone in the circle, everyone turns around, turning his back to the center of the circle. This exercise is designed to help group members focus on the idea of rejection, in terms of both rejecting and being rejected. Another example is having group members divide up into pairs. They sit on the floor, facing each other. Partner A closes his eyes and partner B touches A's face in any way that he likes for a few minutes. The roles are then reversed. This exercise is designed to focus on the idea of touching and of being touched and on the different kinds of touching.

The format for this type of group usually alternates between doing an activity and talking about the feelings and ideas that were aroused by the activity. One example is a group whose activity is creating murals. At the beginning of each meeting of the group, a large piece of paper is hung on the wall. Group members sit in front of the paper, on couches, or on the floor. A table with different kinds of paint and media for drawing is placed to the side of the paper. There is minimal group discussion and no preplanning. One group member spontaneously goes to the paper and begins to draw or paint; others join him. The mural may evolve into one picture or into a series of individual pictures. When everyone finishes, they sit together and talk. Group members talk about what they drew or painted, why they created what they did, what it means to them, how it makes them feel, what they were trying to say, and so forth. Other group members tell the patient how they feel about his painting or drawing, what it reminds them of, why they think the patient drew what he did, and so forth. The group explores why they spontaneously created a winter scene together, for example, or why everyone went off on his own and did an individual picture. Interpersonal responses are discussed, such as, what Jane felt when Sue extended her boat to cover part of Jane's abstract design, or what Philip thought when Frank teased him about his funny-looking rabbit and why Frank teased Philip. Sometimes, when a group member says that he feels his drawing was an attempt to express an emotion, idea, need, or value, he is asked if he would like to learn to express that particular aspect of himself more directly. If he says yes, other group members help the patient learn to do this. When the group feels they have talked enough, they begin another mural. It may be done in the same spontaneous way the first mural was done, or the group may decide to do a mural that expresses some theme or idea that had been raised in the previous group discussion.

The purpose of this type of group is to develop cooperative group-interaction skill. The purpose is not awareness and alteration of the many different emotions, responses, and values that are interfering with need satisfaction. This aspect of treatment will be discussed in Chapter 10. In a group designed for learning cooperative group skill, patients are helped to enjoy the experience of being with each other on an emotional level, and how to interact at this level of interpersonal relations in a group situation. There is no attempt to "get it all together," nor is there any lengthy discussion of ineffective patterns of behavior.

The other type of pure group designed to develop cooperative group-interaction skill is one in which the therapist serves primarily as an advisor. She may initially play a relatively active role in the formative period of the group, but later withdraws to a peripheral position. In this position, she is available to the group for consultation and assistance, but she does not participate in their day-to-day, on-going interaction. The formation of the group may be formal or informal. In a formal group, the therapist brings together a number of patients who are ready to begin learning cooperative group-interaction skill and who share some common interests or characteristics. For example, they may all be interested in some aspect of gardening or be of approximately the same age. The common interest should not be so important to group members that they spend most of their time involved in actualization of the interest. For example, a group formed around an interest in photography may spend so much of their time together taking, developing, and printing pictures that they never attend to the intimate, personal aspects of themselves or others. Ideally, the interest is sufficiently general so that there is no end product or goal to be arrived at.

In this learning group brought together in a formal manner, the therapist introduces the participants and emphasizes that their being together is to have fun, to enjoy each other, to share. The idea is to go off together and do whatever they want. After helping the group get started, the therapist, in essence, stays home. Group members know that their advisor-therapist is available if the group as a whole wants to talk about something that is happening in the group or if individual members want to talk. As an example of the former, one group became concerned about Nancy. Everything had been going well until Nancy decided, for no apparent reason, that the group did not want her to be with them any more. The therapist brought Nancy and the other group members together. She helped the group examine what had been happening around the time Nancy decided she was not wanted. What was the group doing that made Nancy feel rejected? Or had Nancy misperceived events taking place in the group? An individual group member may want to talk about how he feels about another group member or about his idea that the group is, for example, demanding he take more responsibility than he is willing to accept. The therapist tries to bring the individual problems of group members back to the group, helping to find ways to solving problems in interaction together.

When a cooperative group is formed in an informal manner, a number of patients spontaneously begin to interact as a group. They break off from some larger group, form a clique, and go off together and "do their own thing." They spend a lot of time together, often in the wider community. The therapist, so to speak, adopts the group, aiding them in their desire to be together and letting them know she is available for help with any problems that may arise. The formation of these spontaneous groups occasionally causes concern to other staff members. They feel that the formation of cliques or splinter groups weakens the larger group, making it less effective as a learning situation. Or, they may feel that any clique is automatically going to be detrimental to the members: Participants will have a negative influence on each other. Although splinter groups detrimental to the learning of group members do occasionally develop, this should not usually be the first thought of the therapist. Rather, the therapist should look at each group member and what the group members seem to be doing together to determine how and why the clique formed. When most of the group members are ready to or have already begun to learn cooperative group skills and if the atmosphere of the group is such that it contributes to skill learning, the therapist encourages and protects the formation of the clique. The spontaneous development of a group devoted to the learning of cooperative group skill is, in a sense, more "natural" than the formal group discussed above. It is more similar to what occurs in the normal developmental process. Group members tend to be less conscious of their learning about how to express emotions and satisfy needs. However, this in no way seems to interfere with the learning process.

Groups devoted to the development of cooperative group-interaction skill tend to be time-limited and closed. That is, the group is formed, there may be some initial movement of people in and out of the group, but from that time on the membership of the group remains fairly stable. Continual movement of people in and out of this type of group is not conducive to learning. Group members must have a strong feeling of togetherness in order to share intimate feelings. Continuous change in group membership limits the possibility of the group developing this sense of group identity. The group ceases to exist when most members have developed the ability to participate in a cooperative group, or have found other community-based groups in which they are able to continue to learn this skill. The group tends to dissolve in rather a spontaneous manner; members move out of the group as they no longer feel a need for the group. The few group members left usually are helped to move into another cooperative skill learning group that is just being formed.

Another way a therapist may help a patient learn how to participate in a cooperative group is to help him locate an appropriate group outside the treatment center. This may be somewhat difficult in that most of the community-based groups of which the therapist is usually aware are primarily task-oriented. However, some places such as church-sponsored organizations, community centers, and senior citizens' clubs may have groups formed primarily for and mostly concerned with bringing people with common interests together. These groups often give little emphasis to accomplishing a particular task. Thus, they may be suitable for learning cooperative group-interaction skill. Involvement in almost any community program may give the patient an opportunity to join an informal group. This would be similar to the formation of a spontaneous group mentioned previously. The therapist gives the patient encouragement, support, and advice while he is moving into a community-based group. The patient knows the therapist is available to him for any type of assistance he may need while he is in the group.

There are some problems in teaching cooperative group skill in a middle-range group. The patient may be encouraged to identify and fulfill the safety and love and belonging needs of other group members. Similarly, he may be helped to identify and express his own needs. However, there may be people in the group who are unable to meet these needs. Therefore, the patient must learn to be selective in terms of whom he turns to for need satisfaction. This makes the learning somewhat more difficult. Reinforcement may be given for expressing emotions and sharing personal feelings. But, again, some group members may not be ready for learning in these areas; there tends to be a lack of reciprocation. Middle-range groups tend to be task-oriented, open-ended in the sense of people moving in and out of the group relatively frequently, and usually only fairly cohesive. All of these factors impede the development of a strong feeling of liking and trust, which is necessary for the sharing of very personal aspects of the self.

Ability to Participate in a Mature Group

In a group concerned primarily with learning to participate in a mature group, the therapist acts, as much as possible, like a group member rather than a leader. She takes only those group membership roles that are necessary for the continuation of the group at a particular moment in time. This encourages other group members to see the necessity for various membership roles and gives them an opportunity to experiment with these roles. The therapist and group members offer reinforcement for any appropriate behavior leading to task completion or need satisfaction. Emphasis is placed on maintaining an adequate balance between the task and need fulfillment. A group designed to teach mature group-interaction skills helps a patient integrate his capacity to select, plan, and carry out a group task and his capacity to satisfy his own needs and the needs of others in a group situation. The other new skill learned in this type of group is how to satisfy the needs of group members with whom the individual shares little in common. Thus, the therapist, in selecting group members, tries to have people in the group who have a variety of interests and backgrounds and people who are different in age and sex.

Any activity that allows for or requires a number of people to work together is appropriate for this type of group. The activity may demand a relatively perfect end product or have an inherent time limit for its successful completion. These characteristics of the activity help group members learn to meet needs even when there is a strong demand to attend to the task. However, in the initial period of learning, it is probably best to avoid this added pressure if possible.

A group for the learning of mature group skill tends to be self-conscious. The group periodically stops its on-going activity to examine what is going on in the group. They attempt to determine if necessary task and social-emotional group membership roles are being taken and, if not, what roles need to be taken. Group members may take turns being an observer of rather than a participant in the group. This allows the individual to see how various roles are played. In addition, the group is able to get feedback from someone who is relatively uninvolved in the group's present interaction. The group may take time out to talk about various group membership roles or to experiment with taking roles in role-playing situations.

One area of concern, for both patient and therapist, is the therapist's position as a peer in the group. The therapist must act like a peer, taking no more responsibility or authority than would be expected of other group members. Conversely, the patients must learn to accept the therapist as a peer—not asking her to take more responsibility or deferring to her because she has an authority position in some settings other than this group. Sometimes group members are too dependent on the therapist or request, in subtle ways, that she take more of a leadership role. And sometimes the therapist inadvertently allows group members to be dependent on her or takes a leadership role. A group observer, whether it be one of the group members or an outsider, can often give the group feedback about the role of the therapist. When necessary, group members and the therapist work together to alter the role of the therapist so that she becomes more of a peer.

It is preferable for a patient to learn mature group skill through participation in a group in the wider community. Groups that are functioning at the level of a mature group usually have little difficulty accepting a person who is ready to learn to interact in a mature group. They are usually able to give the feedback and reinforcement necessary for learning. The therapist helps the patient find an appropriate community-based group. She offers support, advice, and encouragement as the patient begins to participate in the new group. The therapist may meet periodically with a group of patients who are involved in learning mature group-interaction skill in various community-based groups. Group meetings are spent in discussing problems that may have arisen in the community-based groups and ways of solving these problems. Role playing of a specific incident that a patient encountered may be used to practice new ways of interacting.

Isolated aspects of mature group-interaction skill can be learned in a middle-range group. However, participation in such a group does not give the patient the true experience of being in a mature group, which is really the best situation for learning. When there is no opportunity to participate in a mature group or a group designed to develop mature group-interacting skills in the treatment center, the therapist and patient usually try to locate an appropriate group in the wider community.

Summary of Group-Interaction Skills

Group-interaction skills can be learned in a group specially designed to help patients develop a specific level of skill and, with special precautions and assistance, in other types of treatment and community-based groups. It is important for the patient's needs to be met by the therapist while he is learning how to interact in a group. This is true until the cooperative group level is reached. At this point, the group takes over the responsibility for meeting needs. Learning of group-interaction skill is enhanced by the availability of good role models, opportunity for experimentation, feedback, and reinforcement. A person learns how to interact in a variety of groups by participating in groups that require increasingly complex ways of interacting.

SUGGESTED READING

Mosey, Anne. *Three Frames of Reference for Mental Health.* Thorofare, N.J.: Charles B. Slack, 1970, chaps. 5, 7.

CHAPTER 9

DEVELOPMENT OF FACETS
OF THE PUBLIC SELF

After a patient has learned the fundamentals of how to perform a task and participate in a group situation, he is ready to focus on facets of the public self. However, learning in the area of activities of daily living may occur prior to this time. Simple activities of daily living may be used as a means of developing basic skills. Conversely, the more advanced levels in the area of intimacy are more easily learned after the patient has acquired or is ready to acquire the ability to participate in a cooperative group. The kind of job a person is likely to be able to hold and the type of recreational activities in which he is likely to participate are determined, to a great extent, by his level of task and group-interaction skill.

ACTIVITIES OF DAILY LIVING

At the time of initial evaluation or at some later period in the treatment process, the therapist and patient determine what, if any, activities of daily living the patient needs to learn. The learning of activities of daily living begins with an activity the patient feels is of particular importance to him at the present time. For example, he may want to be able to go to the hospital canteen to buy refreshments, but he does not know such things as: Do you ask the sales person to get an item or do you pick it up yourself and bring it to the cashier? How do you figure out if you have received the right change from the cashier? When the patient is unable to say what activity of daily living he would like to learn, the therapist starts either with a simple activity or with an activity that will make life easier for the patient or someone else. For example, when a patient does not know how to take care of his bedroom in the hospital, learning may begin by helping the patient to hang his clothes on hooks and put his underwear and socks

137

in a drawer. Making the bed and sweeping the floor are more difficult tasks, which would be taught later. When a patient is unable to get to the day treatment center by himself and must be brought by a family member, teaching may begin in this area. Traveling to and from the center is complex, but learning in this area helps the patient to be more independent and saves time for the family member.

Ideally, the learning of activities of daily living takes place in the expected environment of the patient. For example, Duane, who is receiving treatment at a day center, does not know how to use an automatic washer and drier. Rather than taking him to the in-patient psychiatric ward to practice using the washer on the ward, learning is directed toward the community. The therapist helps Duane to find a Laundromat in his neighborhood, get his dirty clothes together and sort them if necessary, read the directions at the Laundromat, put the right amount of soap in the machine, determine how to get the right coins to put in the machine, and so forth. At times, initial learning may take place in the treatment center and be followed by practice in the community. For example, Joyce could not mend or alter her own clothes, or those of her children. She brought some clothes in need of repair to the treatment center and learned how to do such things as sew on buttons, turn up a hem, and put on a patch. Later the therapist helped Joyce buy the tools and materials she would need to mend clothes at home. Joyce was then encouraged to do her mending at home. However, if she was confronted with a mending chore she could not figure out, Joyce knew she could bring it to the center for assistance. As treatment continued, Joyce was helped to learn to follow directions from a book about care and alteration of clothing. She also learned about going to her local tailor for assistance and advice.

In preparing to teach activities of daily living, the therapist analyzes the total activity. She breaks the activity down into its various parts and determines the sequential steps to the activity. This is done both to help the therapist identify what the patient must learn and determine the best way to teach the activity. For example, in order to write a personal letter a person has to have paper and pen, be able to write legibly, decide what to say in the letter and how to say it, obtain an envelope and a stamp, find the right address and zip code, and find a mail box. How the therapist begins to teach this activity depends on the assets and limitations of the patient. The therapist may start by writing a letter based on what the patient says and then help him to learn to go to the post office to buy a stamp and mail the letter. Or, the therapist may start with giving the patient paper, pen, envelope, and stamp and encouraging him to write a letter. Later she encourages the patient to locate a pen or an appropriate piece of paper by himself. Or the patient may not know how to use a telephone book to find an address, or where you can find an out-of-town telephone book.

At times the problem is not that the patient does not know how to perform an activity of daily living. He knows how, but he does not engage in the activity with any degree of frequency. For example, Greg knows full well how to take a bath, but he rarely does so. Cleo is quite capable of cooking meals for herself, but she usually goes to the corner luncheonette for her meals and spends more money than she can afford. The therapist and patient have to investigate why the patient is not performing a necessary activity of daily living. Greg may not bathe frequently because no one ever seemed to care if he was clean; or he may feel that bathing regularly is a middle-class norm and anything middle-class is to be avoided. If Greg does not bathe because no one seems to care if he is clean, other patients in Greg's daily living group can encourage him to bathe regularly. They compliment him each time it is evident that he has taken a bath or shower. If Greg does not bathe because it is middle-class to do so, the therapist and group may try to help him understand that there are minimal standards of cleanliness accepted by the majority of people in the community. If he wishes to be a member of the community, he has to meet these standards. Cleo ate out most of the time because she did not like to eat alone. The other people in the luncheonette counter were better than no one. Group members helped Cleo to ask an acquaintance who lived alone in the same apartment building to share one meal a day with her. It was arranged for Cleo and the other lady to shop together each week for the meals they would eat together, splitting the cost of the food. One week Cleo prepared the meals they shared, the next week it was the other lady's turn.

Some activities of daily living are taught in a one-to-one situation because the problem area is fairly unique. In other words, only one or two patients in the treatment center may be having difficulty with a particular activity of daily living. For example, the therapist may help Clark learn how to read the timetable for the bus he will be taking to work. Another patient taught Madeline how to iron a shirt. However, when several patients have common problem areas, a group setting may be used for learning. For example, there may be a grooming group concerned with such things as how to maintain one's hair in an attractive or at least an acceptable manner, selection and care of clothing, make-up, care of finger and toe nails, and maintaining a reasonable level of neatness and cleanliness. A cooking group may focus on what is a balanced diet, meal preparation, and how to shop in an economical manner. There may be a group that teaches patients enough about automobiles to enable them to do simple repairs and talk intelligently to an automobile mechanic. A community-orientation group is designed for patients who have been hospitalized for several years. Group members go out into the community to learn such things as where various facilities are located, how to use public transportation, how to follow directions to a specific place, how to cross a busy street, and so forth. A bureaucratic systems group helps patients learn something about dealing with large organizations. For example, at various times the group may focus on how to apply for a rent decrease, get a telephone connected, return a purchase to a large store, apply for a driver's license, open a checking account, find a reputable television repair man, and the like.

If at all possible, activities of daily living are learned through actual doing in a real situation. Thus, when the telephone at the day treatment center is out of order, a patient who does not know how to report an out-of-order phone to the telephone company is given help in carrying out the task. When the sink stops up, a patient who has never taken care of this type of problem is assisted in solving the problem. Doing is preferable to talking about how to do an activity of daily living. For example, a group of patients may talk about how to order food in a restaurant. But, ideally, this is only the first step. The group then goes out into the community and orders a meal on several occasions. Whenever possible, activities of daily living are demonstrated prior to the patient practicing the activity. The therapist, for example, may first show the patient how to make a bed or dust a chair before encouraging the patient to try these tasks.

Activities of daily living may seem fairly simple and routine to the therapist. But for the patient who is unable to perform many activities of daily living, this is often a difficult area to master. Thus the therapist must take care to break down the activity into its various parts and be sure the patient has learned all aspects of the activity. Also, the therapist must remember that many activities of daily living take considerable practice before they become a natural part of a person's repertoire of behavior.

WORK

For patients who have few work habits, the ideal treatment situation offers the patient an opportunity to participate sequentially in a work group, a sheltered workshop, a hospital job, or a specially selected community job and to receive the help of a vocational counselor. Of course, a given patient may not need all of these services to develop work habits and to find a suitable job. Patients who have some work habits but need assistance in learning others may not, for example, need to start in a work group. They may begin treatment in a sheltered workshop or hospital job.

Work Groups

A patient is usually ready for a work group when he has the ability to participate in a parallel group and possesses simple task skills. The purpose of a work group is to help a patient understand what kind of behavior is expected in a work situation and to begin developing basic work habits. A work group might make small wooden toys or candles using an assembly-line format, reproduce and collate hospital forms or other printed matter, make the noon meal, or take care of the patient library. The usual atmosphere of the group is business-like and work-oriented. Group members are expected to come on time, stay for the whole period the group meets (usually one and a half to two hours), complete assigned tasks whether or not they enjoy the particular task, dress appropriately, not discuss personal problems unrelated to work, and to enter into casual conversation with fellow workers, but in such a way that it does not interfere with the job at hand. The therapist and group members reinforce all work-related behavior.

The role of foreman or work supervisor is sometimes rotated among the group members who are able to take the responsibility. This helps group members learn to get along with a variety of supervisors. Each patient-foreman will vary somewhat in his way of organizing the task and assigning jobs. Thus, group members learn something about the need to adjust to different styles of supervision. Rotating the job of foreman also allows patients to experience what it is like to be in a supervisory capacity. From that position, they are often better able to understand why they are expected to behave in a certain way in a work situation. For example, Frank often left the work group early. Only after taking the foreman role did he begin to see why his leaving early interfered with getting the job done.

One rule of the work group is usually that the work of the group is not interrupted unless some major crisis develops. When a group member is having some sort of personal problem, the therapist helps him while the work of the group continues. However, if the major portion of the group gets into an argument over, for example, whether the foreman should or should not have rejected Ilga's sandal straps, the group stops its work. Group members get together and talk about what just occurred and decide on a better way to handle the situation. The group then returns to work and tries to put into effect the decisions they have just made.

After the group has finished its work for the day, group members usually meet to discuss problems encountered that day. Group members give each other feedback and encouragement. Different ways of behaving may be discussed or suggested to one of the group members. There may be general discussion of what is or is not acceptable behavior in a work situation or how you know when you have talked to a fellow worker long enough and ought to get back to work.

One of the therapist's responsibilities in the work group is to select the activity and, with the help of the supervisor for the week, to get all the tools and materials needed to carry out the activity. Group members do not participate in selecting and planning the activity because that is not the usual situation in a work setting. The therapist helps the supervisor to organize and plan for each work session and advises him on ways of dealing with problems that arise. While the group is working, the therapist gives individual assistance when it is needed. She may help someone who is having trouble with his part of the task or talk with a group member who is experiencing a personal crisis. And, of course, the therapist offers reinforcement, feedback, and encouragement to all group members.

Sheltered Workshops

When a patient has acquired some very basic work habits and is able to function in a work group with a minimal number of personal crises, he is ready to enter a sheltered workshop program. There are essentially two types of sheltered workshops: those that are part of a large treatment facility and those that are organizationally separate from a treatment facility. A sheltered workshop located in a treatment center takes patients from all units of the center. It is usually large, offers several different kinds of jobs, and pays patients for the work they do. An independent sheltered workshop usually serves clients who have both physical and psychosocial work-related problems, offers different kinds of work experience, and may or may not pay clients for the work they do. There is another characteristic that differentiates sheltered workshops: Regardless of where they are located, some workshops are oriented to providing employment for people who cannot hold a job in a competitive market. Other sheltered workshops are concerned only with helping clients develop work habits. And still other workshops are concerned with teaching specific work skills such as preparation for office work or jobs in the clothing industry. However, many sheltered workshops offer two or all three of these services. The activities therapist is involved primarily with sheltered workshop programs that prepare clients for work in the wider community and programs that offer employment for people who are unable to work in a competitive job market. The latter type of program is not designed to bring about change, however, so we shall concern ourselves here only with sheltered workshop programs designed to help clients develop work habits.

Participation in a sheltered workshop is quite different from being in a work group. There are many more people, the atmosphere is more strongly work-oriented, one is usually required to punch a time clock, there is a definite foreman or work supervisor, and, for the first time, the patient may be paid for his work. The patient's primary therapist or the therapist responsible for his work group orients the patient to the sheltered workshop. She tells him what it is going to be like and what will be expected of him. It is often helpful for the therapist and patient to visit the sheltered workshop together before the patient becomes involved in the program. The therapist is then able to introduce the patient to supervisory staff and other patients currently involved in the program. The patient has an opportunity to "feel out" the situation and find his way around. Such basic things as knowing where the bathroom is located and what the workers wear can add to the patient's sense of security as he moves into a new situation. Movement into a sheltered workshop may require another period of evaluation and filling out forms. The therapist gives whatever support and direct assistance the patient needs during this transition period. A sheltered workshop provides a "real" work situation for the patient. No longer is there either a small, relatively intimate group of fellow workers to know and relate to or a somewhat protective therapist to turn to for allaying personal fears and anxieties. The setting is more regimented, and there are many more demands to be met.

The activities therapist's responsibility in a sheltered workshop may involve evaluation or participation in the teaching-learning process or both. Evaluation is similar in most respects to the procedure outlined in Chapter 6. The therapist and patient must determine, however, what job of those available the patient will take in the sheltered workshop. This decision is based on the patient's interests and his current assets and limitations. As a participant in the teaching-learning process, the therapist reinforces all work-oriented and interpersonal behavior appropriate for a work setting. The therapist in the role of a foreman assigns tasks and, if necessary, demonstrates how to do the task. The foreman makes certain the patient knows how to do his assigned task before leaving him to work independently. Increasing emphasis is placed on accuracy, neatness, and doing the job at the rate that would be expected in the business world.

A foreman in a sheltered workshop usually stays in the role of a work supervisor. He deals only with those problems a foreman working in the wider community would be expected to handle. Another therapist in the sheltered workshop is usually assigned to help the patient with difficulties he might encounter on the job or in other areas of his life. These responsibilities are separated in order to help the patient experience a relatively realistic work setting. When a foreman is overly supportive and willing to talk about personal ideas and feelings, the patient may think this is the way a typical foreman acts. This does not mean, however, that the foreman-therapist takes an authoritarian, "I am only interested in getting the job done" approach. The foreman indicates his interest in the patient as a person and his desire and willingness to help the patient learn to function in a work situation. The work supervisor takes a middle position between the warm, sympathetic role a therapist sometimes takes and the strict, impersonal role of a job foreman.

Depending on the situation, the patient usually has an opportunity to meet either with a group of fellow workers in the sheltered workshop or with a group of patients in his treatment unit who are in the process of developing work habits. These meetings, ideally, take place two or three times a week. The purpose of the meeting is to provide support and reassurance. Patients talk about problems they have encountered on the job and are encouraged to think about other ways they might have dealt with the situation. Group members may offer suggestions or advice. Patients also report on the effect of new behavior they have tried on the job. The expression of feelings and ideas about work in general and the specific work setting of the patient is encouraged. When a patient appears to be misperceiving events in the work situation, the therapist or another patient goes into the work situation to try to find out what is going on. He may talk to the work supervisor or other workers or simply observe the work setting for a period of time. This information is brought back to the group meeting and shared. The group members try to help the patient discover why he was misperceiving events and repeatedly stress the reality of the situation.

Patients in a sheltered workshop often have more difficulty with interpersonal interactions than with the actual performance of an assigned job. They may have problems relating to the work supervisor. Common difficulties are being too dependent and overly compliant or strongly disliking or mistrusting authority figures. Some patients simply do not like having someone else tell them what to do or do not want anyone else to be "the boss." Other interpersonal difficulties center around the patient's relationships with his fellow workers. The patient may be belligerent, argumentative, or act as if he is superior to other workers. Or, on the other hand, the patient may be so shy or preoccupied with his own thoughts that he rarely speaks to a fellow worker. A patient is helped to overcome problems in interpersonal relations by assisting him to identify the expectations of a work setting and how his behavior is contrary to these expectations. More acceptable ways of interacting are suggested to the patient, and he is urged to try out these suggestions. Support and reinforcement are provided by the patient's primary therapist and the work discussion group. As the patient begins to act in a more appropriate manner, he receives reinforcement for the behavior within the work setting rather than from an outside source. The need for outside support gradually decreases.

Hospital Jobs and Specially Selected Community Jobs

When a patient seems to be functioning well in a sheltered workshop, he may be ready to go and look for a job. However, some patients may be hesitant to take this big step or feel for one reason or another that they are not ready for the move into the wider community. When possible, these patients are assigned to a hospital job or a specially selected community job. Patients also may be assigned to these jobs without any experience in a work group or sheltered workshop or directly from a work-group experience. A hospital job is a part- or full-time work assignment in an institution. These jobs may involve working in the mail room, messenger service, staff or patient library, reception desk, kitchen, grounds maintenance department, switchboard, canteen, and so forth. A specially selected community job is a part- or full-time work assignment in a local business. The patient may, for example, work as a cashier, a plumber's helper, a carwash attendant, a schoolroom aide, or a waitress.

The therapist or therapists responsible for the hospital or community job program have to find the jobs. This involves contacting work supervisors in the hospital and employers in the community. The therapist explains the purpose of the program and tries to get the supervisor or employer to want a patient to work in their setting. The therapist may have to help the individual determine how he could make use of the services of a patient. Some supervisors and employers are fearful of working with patients simply because they are patients. These fears and anxieties must be allayed. The success of a job placement program is determined to a great extent by the relationship between the responsible therapist and the supervisors and employers. The therapist keeps in close contact with the supervisor or employer, calling or going to see him at least once a week while a patient is working with him. She inquires about how the patient is doing and gives suggestions and advice about ways of relating to the patient if such advice is sought. The therapist tries to establish a friendly rather than a purely business-like relationship with the employer or supervisor. Even when the employer or supervisor is not currently working with a patient, the therapist stops by for an occasional chat. The work supervisor in a community or hospital job is urged to interact with the patient as he usually does with any person he may supervise. The patient is given the same responsibilities and assignments that would be given to an employee. Conversely, the patient is allowed the usual coffee breaks and the opportunity to work without excessive supervision.

With the therapist's assistance, the patient selects a job from the various positions available at the time. If a patient wants a job that is currently being filled by another patient, he may take a less preferred job until the other job becomes available. The therapist in charge of job placement takes the patient to work the first day and introduces him to his supervisor. It is the supervisor's responsibility to orient the patient to the work setting and the job he will be doing and to introduce him to his co-workers. During the time a patient is in a job placement, the therapist occasionally visits the patient on the job. This is done in an unobtrusive way so as not to single the patient out from among his co-workers. Patients in hospital or community jobs usually belong to a work discussion group similar to the type mentioned in relation to a sheltered workshop.

If a patient wishes to change his job placement assignment, he brings this up in his work discussion group. He gives the reasons for wanting to make the change. The group gives feedback to the patient about whether or not his reasons are appropriate. Some reasonable reasons for a patient wanting to change his job placement are that he feels he is ready for a more challenging job, the job he now has is too repetitive and boring, he wants a job for which he will be paid, he wants to try another job to see if he likes it, he wants a more prestigious job, and the like.

A patient may occasionally have to leave a job either because he is not able to do the work or he cannot get along with his supervisor or co-workers. The therapist and members of the work discussion group provide support and reassurance. The patient and group, together, try to determine what went wrong and what additional skills the patient needs. He may be urged to take another job that is less demanding or to return to the sheltered workshop or work group for additional practice of work habits.

A hospital or community job allows the patient to experience a real work situation. He is able to observe other workers and compare his behavior to their way of working and interacting. The therapist responsible for finding such jobs has assured herself that work-related behavior is rewarded in the work situation. Thus, the patient receives reinforcement for appropriate behavior on the job. When a patient is able to handle a hospital or community job comfortably, he is ready to begin to look for a job or return to a job that has been held open for him.

Beginning Employment

Looking for a job and beginning to work often pose problems with which patients may need help. Many patients have no idea about what type of job they would like. The vocational counselor can be of considerable help in this case. The vocational counselor can tell the patient about different kinds of jobs, give various tests to determine what types of occupations the patient is best suited for, and inform the patient about different training programs. The counselor may give direct assistance in getting a job, or he may help the patient locate a suitable employment agency.

A patient may not know very much about a job or training program that has been suggested for his consideration. Ideally, rather than following the suggestion blindly, the patient is encouraged to get further information before making a decision. In addition to talking to the vocational counselor about the suggested type of work, the patient is advised to seek information in the community. He might be an observer for a period of time in an appropriate work setting or talk to people who are working at the suggested job. When possible, the patient is urged to work in an appropriate work setting in some capacity for a while. For example, Karen was considering studying to become a dental technician. A temporary job as a receptionist for a dentist who employed several dental technicians was found for her. After observing what dental technicians really do, Karen was in a much better position to decide whether or not she wanted to prepare for this type of work.

Many treatment centers have a special discussion group for both patients who are ready to look for a job and patients who have just begun to work. This group may be led by a vocational counselor or activities therapist. Some things talked about in an employment group are: How do you go about looking for a job? What should you bring to a job interview? What kinds of questions will you be asked? What questions should you ask? What do you say about your period of unemployment? What kind of problems can you expect to encounter on the job, and how do you deal with different situations? The group shares their various experiences and gives encouragement and advice as needed. Patients talk about their ideas, feelings, and attitudes to determine whether they are interfering with the possibility of having a good work experience. A patient usually continues to meet with the employment group until he feels able to make it on his own in the working world.

The Work of Homemakers, Parents, and Students

In addition to helping a patient develop skills that will enable him to prepare for or obtain a paying job, the therapist is concerned with the work of homemakers, parents, and students. There are two aspects to each of these work roles. Borrowing terminology used in the discussion of group dynamics, each of these jobs can be divided into task roles and social-emotional roles. Examples of task roles are the homemaker washing windows and doing the grocery shopping, the parent buying clothes and making dental appointments, and the student studying and taking tests. Examples of social-emotional roles are the homemaker trying to maintain a congenial home atmosphere and making time to spend with each family member, the parent disciplining the child and satisfying his needs, and the student trying to get along with his teachers and classmates.

The Work of the Homemaker. The task responsibilities of a homemaker are similar in many respects to the activities of daily living discussed in the last section. The primary difference is that the homemaker takes responsibility for many of the activities of daily living of other people as well as himself. For example, he does the laundry for all family members and he makes everyone's dinner. When a treatment facility is large, there may be a special unit designed to teach basic homemaking task skills. The unit is sometimes laid out like a home with a living room, kitchen, dining room, and bath. A work room equipped to teach sewing and simple household repairs may be nearby. A small treatment center usually has a homemaking group which uses ward facilities for the learning of home-making task skills.

After evaluation, the patient goes to the homemaking unit or joins the homemaking group to begin developing the required skills. Although the patient may initially work with two or three other patients in doing a task, it is important that he learn eventually to do household tasks independently. For example, at the beginning of treatment the patient may go with the therapist and one other patient to buy cleaning supplies. Later, he is encouraged and reinforced for going to the store alone. Household tasks are taught in realistic wholes. For example, rather than just helping a patient learn to dust furniture as an isolated task, this is learned in the context of cleaning a room. Initially, the therapist may have to clean most of the room while the patient dusts the furniture. But later the patient is helped to learn the sequence of tasks involved in cleaning a room.

Logical ordering and simplicity are emphasized in teaching household tasks. Logical ordering refers to thinking a task through before beginning it—deciding what should be done first, what second, and so forth. For example, when do you put soap in the washing machine, or does it take longer to cook the rice or the meat? Simplicity refers to doing tasks in the easiest and least time-consuming manner. It is easier, for example, to clean a floor with a sponge mop than a rag mop, and it takes less time to butter toast when the butter is soft. The patient is introduced to labor-saving devices, fancy cleaning products, and prepared foods only if it is economically feasible for him to use these items in his own home. Saving time is emphasized. For example, it takes less time to clean a bathroom when cleaning supplies are left by the door than if you run to get each item as it is needed. It saves time if you stop by the shoe repair shop on the way to the bakery rather than making a special trip.

Any mechanical household item the patient encounters in the learning situation is studied in detail. For example, if the patient uses a toaster-oven in the process of learning how to cook, he should not only learn what temperatures are used for cooking various foods, but also how to take out the crumb tray and clean the glass door. The patient learns to use a vacuum cleaner, and how to empty the cleaner and insert a new dust bag. And where do you buy dust bags? Simple household repairs are also taught, for example, how to put caulk around the bathtub, hang a curtain rod, prepare a wooden floor for waxing, and level a refrigerator.

Because many homemakers are responsible for family finances, this area is frequently studied in a homemaking group. The group members might go to the grocery store and have the manager explain unit pricing, explore the neighborhood to find out which hardware store has the least expensive plastic pail, study the pros and cons of buying furniture on time, invite an accountant to come and explain how to fill out an income tax form, and find out whether a particular group member is eligible for food stamps.

The teaching of homemaking skills is made to be as personal as possible. Learning is closely related to the individual's own home situation. For example, rather than learning how to prepare a budget by making up one for some hypothetical family, the patient prepares a month's budget for his own family. Similarly, in learning to plan meals the patient plans actual family meals, taking into consideration the likes, dislikes, and nutritional needs of each family member. The learning situation is made as similar as possible to the living situation of the patients who are treated at the center. Economic and ethnic backgrounds are taken into consideration. A fancy, shiny kitchen unit is avoided, for example, in a center located in a low economic area. It is nice to have such a unit, but it does not meet the learning needs of the patient groups. They do not need, for example, to learn how to use an oven with an automatic timer. They may well need to learn how to cope with an oven that heats unevenly. In learning about meal preparation, the patient works with the kinds of foods he and his family like and usually eat. Sometimes ethnic dishes are somewhat difficult to prepare and require special ingredients. But the end result is ultimately more meaningful and rewarding for the patient.

Once the patient has developed some homemaking skills, he is urged to practice these skills in his own home if at all possible. Problems encountered in using skills are then brought back and discussed with the therapist and fellow patients in the homemaking unit or group. By applying skills in his own home, the patient is better able to see what he has learned and what additional skills he needs to acquire. Hopefully the patient receives reinforcement for his new homemaking skills both from other family members and from his own sense of mastery of household tasks. This is important in that it enables the patient to experience the doing of household tasks as rewarding and need fulfilling.

Many patients *have* homemaking task skills. Their difficulty is that they either do not use these skills or spend too much of their time taking care of the home. For example, Millicent knows perfectly well how to cook, clean, and shop for her family. But for the last two months she has spent most of her time sitting in a rocking chair looking out of the window or crying. Conversely, Carl spends all day and most of the evening occupied by household tasks. The reasons for these patterns of behavior may be related to personal problems or problems within the home setting or both. Patients with personal problems would include Arthur, who does almost no household tasks because he feels he should spend all of his time praying, and Zelda, who spends most of her time doing household chores because, if she does not keep very busy, she starts thinking about things she does not want to think about. Joan, who refuses to do household tasks because no one in the family seems to appreciate what she does, and Irene, who feels excluded from the activities of her husband and preadolescent son and therefore avoids them by keeping occupied with household tasks, have family-interaction problems. Some of these problem areas are best dealt with in treatment related to facets of the private self, to be discussed in the next chapter. Family activities therapy, also to be discussed in the following chapter, is ideal for the treatment of many family-related homemaking problems.

However, many difficulties in homemaking, both task and social-emotional, can be best handled in a discussion group. A homemaking discussion group focuses primarily on the question, "Why am I having difficulty in the area of homemaking and what can I do about these difficulties?" The group is concerned with identifying the problem, discovering its immediate source, discussing ways of solving the problem, trying solutions in the family situation and, if that does not work, trying something else. Support, encouragement, and advice are offered as needed. A homemakers' discussion group deals with such typical difficulties as, "No one but me does anything around this house," "I could get a different breakfast for everyone and they would still complain," "I work so hard all day that I'm exhausted when everyone comes home," and "I want some time for myself."

Many of these problem areas boil down to establishing priorities, using time effectively, and getting other family members either to appreciate the job of a homemaker or to share in the doing of household tasks. Some homemakers cannot set priorities: They have no sense of what has to be done, what can wait until later, and what can just be left undone. They need concrete help in looking at all of their household tasks to organize them in terms of their importance to the individual and other family members. Patients who have difficulties establishing priorities also need help in identifying their ideas and feelings about putting off tasks for a later time or not doing some tasks at all. For example, Paul had the idea that all the beds had to be made before leaving for work. He felt that not getting the beds made in and of itself meant that one was not taking care of a home properly. It took some time for Paul to realize that, in reality, this was a ridiculous idea. The world did not cave in if beds were not made. There are sometimes other, more important jobs to be done in the morning.

Some patients have difficulty using time effectively. They seem to be working at household tasks all of the time and yet there always seem to be more chores to do. These homemakers, for example, start washing dishes, stop to watch a news program on television, begin to pick up the living room, remember that there are clothes that need to be brought to the cleaners, start getting the clothes together in a pile, notice a story on the front page of the newspaper, stop to read the story, and so on. They never seem to have time to do the things they enjoy, because the housework never gets done. In a homemakers' discussion group, patients who have problems using time effectively are helped to make up a weekly work schedule. This schedule specifies the time and day for doing various household chores and blocks of free time. The patient is encouraged to follow the schedule, getting tasks done in the allotted time, completing each task before starting another, not doing something else when the schedule indicates she should be working, and using free time doing something she enjoys. Having and using scheduled free time often serves as a reinforcer. Group members offer praise and compliments for following the schedule. Nonadherence to the schedule is examined to determine the immediate cause and what the patient might do in order to follow the schedule more closely.

Family members sometimes take a homemaker's work for granted. They show little appreciation for what is being done to make their life more comfortable. Thus, the homemaker receives little reinforcement for his work, except perhaps a sense of satisfaction derived from maintaining a pleasant home. This type of satisfaction only goes so far; most homemakers need some appreciation and thanks from family members. When one or more members of the homemaking discussion group have difficulty in this area, the group tries to think of ways one can obtain recognition for adequate maintenance of the home. For example, the homemaker might ask directly for appreciation, or not do some household tasks and wait for family members to realize how important these tasks are for their well-being, or insist that other family members do some household task for a period of time so they can acquire some idea of the time and energy spent on the task. The patient is urged to try out a suggested course of action and report back to the group. When one way of dealing with the problem does not work, the patient is encouraged to try another solution. The group provides support and reinforcement as the patient tries to alter his home situation.

Homemakers sometimes have the idea that they alone are responsible for doing all household tasks. As a result, they never indicate to family members that help would be appreciated. They may even indicate that they do not want any assistance. The homemaker ends up playing the role of a martyr or household drudge or he is completely exhausted. If a patient has difficulty in this area, the homemaking discussion group, when necessary, first helps the patient realize that he is not requesting family members to share household tasks. The ideas that support this manner of behaving are examined. For example, the patient's whole sense of identity may rest on being a homemaker, or he may feel that he is not as good as other family members and household tasks should be performed by inferior people, or he cannot do anything other than household chores. The fallacy of these usually unconscious ideas is exposed. More realistic ideas about the self in relation to others are suggested. The patient is urged both to take over these suggested ideas and to act on the basis of this new way of thinking about himself. For example, Lynn felt her husband would refuse if she asked for help around the house. The group urged Lynn to try asking for help. How to request help was practiced in role playing. Lynn was reminded to ask directly and to specify what tasks she wanted her husband to do. She tried this. Her husband grudgingly did a few chores but was not very pleasant about it. Lynn told the group what had happened. They complimented her on her efforts, told her to ignore the unpleasantness, and to praise her husband for everything he did. She was urged to continue requesting help, and it was suggested that she ask her husband to do chores that would allow them to spend more time together. Through the support and suggestions of the group, Lynn was able to get the help she wanted.

The Work of a Parent. The work of a homemaker and the work of a parent often overlap and intermingle. However, some patients have no difficulties in the area of homemaking, but do have problems with child rearing. When this is a common problem area for patients at the treatment center, there may be an on-going parents' discussion group at the center. This is usually a mixed group of both men and women. Sometimes the group is open to anyone in the community who wants help with being a parent, or the spouse of the patient may be invited to join the group. Ideally, the group is co-led by a male and a female therapist who have had some experience in raising a child. According to the needs of members, the group may discuss any number of aspects of being a parent: How often should you take a child to the dentist? What can you do if a child refuses to go to bed? How do you teach a child to pick up after himself? Is a particular child really afraid to go to school alone, or is this a way of getting special attention? Should siblings fight out their own battles without parental intervention? When should a child be able to use the family car? Guest speakers, such as a nutritionist, a child psychologist, a parole officer, or the director of a local settlement house, may be invited occasionally.

Group members are urged to share their feelings and anxieties about child rearing. Stereotypes of the "good parent" are avoided, for example, the myths that a good mother immediately loves her child at birth or that a good parent is always consistent. It is emphasized that occasional feelings such as hostility, anger, disappointment, of being overwhelmed by the job, or resentment that a child is interfering with one's life are normal reactions and not a sign an individual is not a proper parent.

Chronic negative reactions are accepted by the group as a problem that they will try to help the individual resolve. The parent is assisted in examining his ideals, values, and life situation to determine what is interfering with his developing a positive parent-child relationship. For example, Beverly, a young mother, felt overwhelmed by the task of caring for three children under the age of four. She had no husband, could not afford a baby sitter, and had no friends. With the support of the group and the help of another group member, Beverly was able to enroll the oldest child in a city-supported day care center. With further encouragement, Beverly joined a cooperative baby-sitting group in her neighborhood. Through participating in this group, Beverly was able to gain some free time away from the children, and she also developed a friendly relationship with a few of the co-op group members. With these community-based supports, Beverly felt much less harried and pressured by her child-rearing responsibilities. Another example is Elliot, who constantly argued with his twelve-year-old son. He did not like his son's friends, the kinds of activities he engaged in after school, his grades in school, the clothes he wore, and so forth. Elliot said he was sure the boy was going to grow up and be like his stepbrother, who was currently in jail. There was no evidence, however, that the son was going to get into trouble. After considerable discussion it was discovered that Elliot felt it was a sign of disrespect each time his son did something against his wishes. To Elliot a difference in opinion with his son was a personal insult. When Elliot could get his son to do something he wanted him to do, he felt strong and in control. When the son did what he wanted to do, Elliot felt insignificant. It was further discovered that Elliot had no way of satisfying his need of mastery. He was using his son for this purpose. The group repeatedly emphasized to Elliot that he was a respected member of the community and gave him affection and attention. Elliot's ideas about the father-son relationship were clarified, and Elliot was told about a twelve-year-old boy's need to make many of his own decisions. The group encouraged Elliot to stop arguing with his son. When he became angry about a decision his son had made, he was told not to say anything to his son. Rather, he should vent his angry feelings in the group and tell them about the incident. When Elliot did this, the group examined the incident and gave Elliot feedback about his son's decision or behavior. They reassured Elliot that his son respected him. Elliot was also helped to find ways of satisfying his need for mastery. After attempting several activities, Elliot finally joined a rifle club where he learned about guns and how to shoot. Slowly Elliot was able to give his son more independence, and their relationship improved markedly.

One thing emphasized in the parents' discussion group is being truly *with* a child. Some parents have difficulty doing things with their children. They seem to have lost the ability to play. Often, they themselves engage in few recreational activities. One way of helping a patient with difficulty in this area is to have him and another group member who is able to play, and has a child of about the same age, plan activities they can do together with their children. Through participation in these activities, the parent is able to get some idea about what a parent-child play relation is like. He may be able to use the other group member as a model. For a parent with young children, the therapist or another group member may go into the home and play with the children. The parent is encouraged to observe and participate. Hopefully, the parent will receive reinforcement from both the pleasure of play itself and the pleasurable reaction of his child.

The Work of a Student. Finally, the last area of work to be discussed is the work of a student. A student must be able to study, take tests, and get along with his teachers and classmates. Ideally, these areas of difficulty are dealt with in a school setting. A large treatment center often has a school program with specially trained teachers to help the students. Or the patient may go to a school in the community which is designed to help students who have psychological problems. When these special facilities are available, the primary therapist serves as a liaison between the school and the treatment unit and coordinates the school program with the patient's other learning experiences.

If there is no school facility, the activities therapist may take over this aspect of the treatment. Problems in authority-teacher relationships can be dealt with fairly easily in a work group or sheltered workshop program. Although these learning settings are somewhat different than a school, there is enough similarity to allow for learning. Through reinforcement and feedback, the work supervisor helps the patient relate to authority in an acceptable manner. Difficulties in relating to classmates can also be dealt with in work-oriented settings as well as in task and egocentric-cooperative groups. The treatment process is similar to the one discussed for learning how to get along with fellow workers or group members, so it will not be repeated here.

Helping a patient learn how to study may involve a one-to-one interaction between therapist and patient. They work together to identify problem areas and ways of solving these problems. For example, when the problem is one of concentration, the patient may be encouraged to study for a short period of time. If he actually studies for this period, he receives some kind of reinforcement. The period of time for study is gradually increased until the patient is studying approximately the same amount of time he would be required to study if he were going to school. For another patient, the problem might be being able to pick out what is important to learn and what is irrelevant. Using the patient's usual textbooks, the therapist first goes over several lessons, showing the patient the significant ideas to be learned. Later the patient is urged to select important items. The therapist provides considerable feedback and corrects any errors the patient may make.

A similar technique is used in helping the patient learn how to take tests. For example, if a patient has difficulty with essay tests, the therapist may give him a reading assignment followed by an essay test which she has prepared. The therapist and patient go over the completed test together, identifying areas of difficulties. The therapist suggests other ways the patient might deal with the material. Another reading assignment is given, and the process is repeated until the patient has grasped the essentials of taking essay tests. In another instance, the problem may be anxiety related to tests. Treatment may start by giving the patient a test that will be easy for him to complete successfully. The consequences of getting a failing grade are mild, such as not being able to have dessert with lunch. Gradually the tests are made more difficult and the consequences of failing more severe. This is a gradual method of helping the patient learn to live with the pressures of taking tests.

When a student is having trouble with a particular school subject or is not at his grade level in a subject, the therapist may tutor the patient or find someone else who can do this. Another patient may act as tutor, or someone from the community may be invited to help. Many schools and youth organizations have groups of young people who are willing and prepared to act as tutors. This is usually a voluntary service. When possible, tutoring is done in the community rather than in the treatment center. This gives the patient one more opportunity to be a participant in the community.

When a patient has solved a fair number of his problems of being a student, he is usually urged to go back to his regular school or to the local community school. The patient is given support and encouragement and an opportunity to discuss any problems he may encounter. The therapist either suggests or helps the patient discover for himself a way of solving the problem. This is tried in school and the patient and therapist decide if the solution was effective and need gratifying for the patient. If it was not a successful solution, the patient tries another way of solving the problem. On occasion, the therapist may, with the patient, visit his teachers to discuss his progress. When there are several students at the treatment center who are attending school, a student discussion group may be formed. This group would be similar to the other work-related discussion groups described in this chapter.

Many activities therapists have had little experience in the area of education. Thus, they may find it difficult to help a patient with some school problems. It may be helpful for the therapist to read about such subjects as "how to study" and test construction. Observation in a classroom is particularly useful. The therapist may on occasion find assistance through consultation with a school teacher. The teacher consulted may be one of the patient's usual instructors, or he may be a teacher who has had some experiences in dealing with problems similar to those of the patient.

Summary

This rather lengthy section on treatment in the area of work has emphasized the dual aspects of work. The ability to work includes both being able to do particular tasks and being able to form good relationships with other people in the work situation. Work habits are best acquired through interaction in a work setting or a simulation of a work situation. Ideally, there is an opportunity to experience work difficulties, talk about these difficulties, and actively attempt to overcome the problems of interacting in a work setting. The length of this section is probably indicative of the importance of work for most people in our society. To them, work is a significant source of need satisfaction and a large factor in their sense of identity.

RECREATION

In assessing the area of recreation, the therapist and patient attempt to determine whether the recreational aspects of the patient's life are a source of satisfaction for him. Common problems in the area of recreation are not putting aside sufficient time for recreation, a value system that places a negative value on recreation, insufficient knowledge of recreational facilities, and lack of recreational skills. Patients may have one or several of these problems.

Many treatment centers have a recreational group designed to deal with general problems in the use of free time. This is usually both a discussion and activities group. As an activities group it may try various recreational activities together, such as playing pool, participating in a touch football game, going out to dinner or a movie together, visiting a local street fair, and so forth. After participating in the recreational activity or the next day, the group discusses their feelings and ideas about the activity. Was it enjoyable, and what made it so? What needs were satisfied? What emotions were experienced? What made the activity disappointing? Is this something that might be enjoyed with other people?

The purpose of this group is both to help members test whether they enjoy various recreational activities and to identify and alter ideas, feelings, and values that interfere with enjoyment of recreational activities. Becky, for example, had never given any consideration to what recreational activities she liked or disliked. She lived within a close-knit family group who jointly decided on recreational activities in which everyone was expected to participate. No one asked Becky what she would like to do. During initial involvement in the recreational group, Becky was encouraged to participate in the activity selected by the group. However, after participation, she was helped to discover how she had felt: Was it fun or wasn't it? And what was there about the activity she had enjoyed and what was unpleasant? Through this experience, Becky began both to realize that she had a right to enjoy recreational activities and to identify the things she liked to do. Later in her involvement in the recreational group, Becky was helped to tell the group what activities she wanted to do and to persuade them to join her in the activity. This was done to assist

Becky in developing the skills she would need to get her family group to recognize her interests and to share recreational activities that met her needs.

A recreational group also emphasizes the use of free time independent from group activities. Group members are encouraged to plan evening and week-end recreational activities. The group helps individuals decide what they are going to do and assists each person in carrying out planned activities. For example, Edgar decided to spend Saturday afternoon browsing in used book stores. But it was rainy that Saturday, so Edgar stayed home watching television programs he did not particularly enjoy. On the following Monday, he told the group he did not visit book stores because it had rained. This was a typical pattern for Edgar: He would plan a recreational activity, but there was always something that inter-fered. After Edgar and the group talked about this pattern, it was decided that Edgar should call another group member when he found some reason for not doing a planned activity. At first, Edgar did not want to do this because he was afraid to disturb anyone with his problems. With continued encouragement, he began to call a group member. As planned, this person went to Edgar's apartment and joined him in whatever recreational activity he had decided to do. The anticipated pleasure in participating in recreational activities was finally so great that Edgar came to realize that his excuses for not doing things he enjoyed were rather ridiculous. He was ultimately able to pursue activities he enjoyed without the assistance of a group member.

Sometimes, patients have little awareness of the recreational activities available in the community. A recreational group often assigns itself the task of investigating recreational facilities in the community. This may involve going to such places as a "Y," settlement house, church, or museum to find out what types of programs they have for members or the general public. Or some group members may go through the newspaper to find notices of available recreational activities. Other group members may get information from the city's visitors bureau or the state tourist information center. This information is shared with fellow group members and often posted for the benefit of other persons in the treatment center.

Group members give each other encouragement and support in engaging in these newly identified recreational activities. Any problems encountered are brought back to the group for discussion. For example, Diana decided to take an evening oil painting course at the local high school.

After going to the first session she told the group she had decided not to take the course. She said the other students were unfriendly and talked only to each other. No one had paid any attention to her. Diana was helped to understand that she had to make an effort to talk to the other students, that people were not going to act friendly unless she approached them in a friendly manner. The group participated in role-playing situations with Diana. Diana was able to act out various ways of making friendly overtures to a stranger. She was encouraged to go to another class meeting and try out some of these approaches. With support from the group, Diana was able to attend classes and form casual relationships with her fellow classmates. Eventually, she was able to get sufficient pleasure from the class meetings that she no longer needed reinforcement from the group.

At times, difficulties in the area of recreation are dealt with on a one-to-one basis. The therapist and patient talk about possible activities the patient might enjoy. Knowing the community, the patient's assets and limitations, and the patient's financial situation, the therapist suggests only those activities in which the patient is likely to be able to participate after he leaves the treatment center. The point is to help the patient find future recreational activities, not just something to occupy his time in the present situation. When a patient has no idea about what activities he might enjoy, the therapist encourages him to try a variety of different activities. If there are special-interest, recreation-oriented groups in the treatment center, the patient is urged to join some of these groups on a trial basis. There is usually an arts and crafts room where the patient can try out various activities alone or with the help of the therapist. The therapist and patient may try playing various games such as chess or pool and sports activities. When the patient finds an activity he enjoys, the therapist helps him develop beginning skill in the activity. After the patient has learned the basics, he and the therapist find some place in the community where he can continue to participate in the recreational activity. For example, Ryan helped some patients make silk-screen greeting cards in the arts and crafts room, and decided that he would like to do silk screening. He and the therapist borrowed instruction books from the local library and together practiced the basic steps of silk screening. Ryan learned how to make a screen, cut and apply the film, and print multicolored images. When Ryan felt secure in the basic steps, the therapist encouraged him to contact several organizations to find out if they had any groups involved with silk screening. Finally, Ryan found a church group that was responsible for church publicity. They had never used silk screening for making posters and notices for meetings but thought they might like to try this method of reproduction. With the therapist's initial support, Ryan joined the group. Regardless of whether the recreational activity is one that is usually done in one's home, the therapist tries to help the patient locate other people in the community with similar interests. This provides both a source for help with the activity and the opportunity to make friends.

In helping a patient develop recreational interests, the therapist looks at all aspects of a recreational activity. Each aspect of the activity is analyzed so that both the patient and therapist are aware of what needs to be learned. For example, to play softball a person has to know how to throw, catch, and bat a ball, and the rules of the game. He must know how to cooperate with teammates and engage in friendly competition with the other team. In addition, the person must be able to locate and join a softball team or get together a group of people who want to play softball.

The community activities aspect of recreation is emphasized in many treatment centers. This is particularly true when the center is in and serves a designated community. Community members are often invited to the treatment center to talk about the activities in which they are involved. They are able to outline the needs of the community and to help patients become aware of ways in which they can contribute to the community. The recreational group mentioned previously may devote much of its attention to helping patients to learn how to engage in community activities, or there may be another group concerned exclusively with this aspect of recreation. A community activities group is usually a discussion group. In other words, the group as a whole does not participate in a community activity; rather, group members are encouraged to join in community activities of their choice. For example, various group members may be involved in such activities as acting as a volunteer receptionist at the local hospital, stuffing envelopes in the campaign headquarters of a political candidate, joining a group that is planning a demonstration for better street lights, or visiting older people who are unable to leave their homes.

The purpose of the community activities group is to acquaint patients with possible ways of serving the community and to help them develop the skills they will need for community service. A new patient in the group is told about some community activities and is helped to decide what he is able to do and the kinds of activities he would enjoy. Often a patient will join in a community activity with another group member for a period of time. The other patient is able to provide support and give the patient direct assistance in the situation. Later, the patient is urged to join in a community activity of his own. This gives him an opportunity to learn how to become part of a community group and to participate independent of the help of another patient. Group members discuss problems they have encountered in their community activity. As in other discussion groups, they help each other develop more useful patterns of interaction.

Patients with difficulty in the area of recreation are helped to develop as many recreational interests as possible. The more interests a person has, the more likely he is to find ways of satisfying his needs. Patients are given assistance in identifying needs that are not being met in other aspects of their life. They are helped to look at recreational activities in terms of what possible needs an activity can satisfy. For all patients, the emphasis is on finding activities they can enjoy. For that, after all, is the purpose of recreation.

INTIMACY

Intimacy is the area of human experience that involves a close, sustained relationship with other individuals. It is a facet of man that appears to be acquired in stages in the normal developmental process. Thus, it is taught in stages in the treatment process. The patient is helped to develop his ability to engage in intimate relationships to the extent that he is able to acquire this ability. Some patients are only able to get to the point of forming casual friendships. Others, however, are able to go on to the point of developing love or nurturing relationships.

Casual Relationships

A person usually learns how to make friends by having friendly people with common interests available and by observing how friends interact. Some patients have no idea how to go about making friends. They do not know how to talk to another individual, how to ask someone to do something with them, how a friend usually behaves, and so forth. In helping a patient make friends, the therapist often needs to talk with the patient about what is involved in making and keeping friends. The patient is urged to spend time with other people who have interests similar to his own. These may be fellow patients, acquaintances in the community, or people in some sort of community agency or center. He is particularly urged to spend time with other people outside the context of an organized activity. For example, the patient is encouraged to eat lunch with another patient or to ask a person in the ceramics group he attends at the community center to go to a movie with him. The therapist offers support, advice, and reassurance, and attempts to arrange things so the patient receives some sort of reinforcement for friendly interactions. This external reinforcement may be necessary until the patient is able to get some degree of need satisfaction from his interactions with others.

To facilitate the formation of casual friendships, the therapist may suggest the patient do a specific task with another patient who has similar interests. She may suggest, for example, that they play some game together or go shopping. The task suggested should be well within the abilities of both patients, so they do not become preoccupied with the task. This allows for more attention to personal interaction. The therapist might have to suggest shared tasks for some period of time before the individuals begin to do things together spontaneously.

People also learn about friendships by observing how friends interact. Thus, friendships between patients in the treatment center are encouraged, giving patients an opportunity to see friendship in action. The staff members also serve as models. Ideally, staff members allow their casual, friendly interactions to be evident to patients. They do not save the showing of affection, kidding around, and mild teasing just for the staff room or after-hours interactions. The patients should be allowed to see the staff as a group of friendly co-workers.

Chum Relationships

It is more difficult to help a patient develop a chum relationship than casual relationships. The partner in a chum relationship must be someone who is also at the point of needing and wanting a chum relationship. The therapist and patient seek out a situation in which the patient is likely to find someone with whom he can form a chum relationship. The most likely situation is one in which there are people who have backgrounds and interests similar to those of the patient. Once a group of like-minded individuals is found, the patient is encouraged to join in their activities.

A patient who has never been in a chum relationship is often fearful of any degree of intimacy. He may be afraid he will become too dependent if he lets himself get involved with another person, or lose his sense of individual identity. Dependency and some loss of individual identity are part of a chum relationship. The patient may need reassurance that these experiences are not destructive, but rather essential for growth in this area.

As with all aspects of treatment, the therapist can only design learning situations and offer support. The patient must do the learning. When a patient does begin to form a chum relationship, he may or may not want to talk about the relationship with the therapist. There is a degree of secrecy in a chum relationship. Thus, the patient may want to develop this relationship independent of the therapist's direct assistance. The therapist does not question the patient about the relationship. She is able to help the patient by giving approval of the relationship and making whatever arrangements are needed so the patient is able to spend time alone with his friend.

Love Relationships

As with a chum relationship, a therapist can only help the patient find other people with whom he might form a love relationship. The therapist provides support and advice when it is requested, and reassures the patient that he has the capacity to form love relationships. It is important for the therapist to feel and communicate a sense of satisfaction that the patient is moving into relationships from which she is excluded. One situation that particularly encourages the development of love relationships is communal living outside a family setting. The give and take and closeness required in sharing household tasks and the need for mutual need satisfaction often facilitates the growth of love relationships. Therefore, if the patient's life situation permits, the therapist may help him to find some sort of communal living arrangement.

Nurturing Relationships

In the normal developmental process a person learns to be the nurturing partner in a relationship first by participating in a relationship in which he is the nurtured partner. A man, for example, learns something about being a father from being a son. Other events that contribute to learning are observation of various nurturing relationships, caring for a garden or some kind of animal, and being given partial responsibility for the care of another person. The activities therapist uses this information about normal development as the basis for designing learning situations for development of the ability to nurture.

This aspect of intimacy is usually learned toward the end of the treatment process. Thus, the patient has recently experienced the role of the nurtured partner. He is able to draw on this experience as he begins to consider what he must do in the role of the nurturing partner. The patient may be encouraged to buy an animal or some plants as a way of trying out this role. In caring for these objects, the patient is able to experience what it is like to spend time and energy taking care of something other than himself. Feelings aroused by having something be dependent upon oneself and the need, at times, to put aside other interests and concerns can also be experienced. The therapist helps the patient to express these feelings and to understand that they are a normal part of the nurturing process. Dealing with such practical matters as getting someone to care for his dog, if the patient is to be away for the weekend, and how one finds out when African violets should be transplanted, also gives the patient an idea of other aspects of the nurturing process.

Later, the patient may be given responsibility for helping another patient. This may involve assisting a new patient to unpack his clothes, get settled in his room, and discover the physical layout and rules of the ward. Or the patient may work as a volunteer in a child day care center or in the playroom of a hospital pediatric ward. The therapist gives the patient support and encourages him to talk about the experience. Discussion is focused on required tasks as well as on the emotional aspects of the relationship. The patient, for example, is given help in deciding what initial rules and norms he should tell the new patient in addition to how to give this information. Such matters as how to express affection, show approval, allay anxiety, and fulfill safety needs are discussed in detail.

When a patient is having difficulty giving nurturence to his own child or children, it is sometimes useful to bring the child into the treatment center. The child may be brought to the center several afternoons a week or spend the weekend if the patient is in the hospital full time. Some in-patient treatment centers have facilities so that children may stay with their parent all the time. There may be a nursery, several small apartments, or the child may stay in his parent's room. In a day treatment center, the parent may bring the child with him in the morning or arrange to have him come after school. Some treatment centers have a child day care center for the children of both patients and staff members.

The parent is usually given considerable help in caring for his child at first. This is done for three reasons. Patients who have difficulty in caring for their children often come to the center with a profound sense of being overwhelmed by the task. They are exhausted from their struggle to deal with the demands of child rearing and from the need to control their negative feelings. With someone else taking over some of the responsibility, they are first able to relax and feel some degree of freedom. Another reason for giving considerable assistance is to place the patient in a position from which he is able to view the situation with some degree of perspective. The parent is given help in discovering what the problems are and how these problems might be solved. The parent is also urged to express his feelings and to examine his ideas about the nurturing relationship. He is encouraged to test the reality or reasonableness of his ideas. The third reason the parent is initially given considerable help in caring for his child is that this gives him an opportunity to observe someone else in a nurturing role. He is able to see, for example, how another person fulfills his child's esteem needs and deals with his poor eating habits.

Very gradually, the parent is urged to take increasing responsibility for the child. He is encouraged to spend more time with the child, first in the company of others and later with the child alone. Feedback and support are freely given, as is advice when it is requested. The parent is helped to identify the needs of the child and to experiment with ways of meeting these needs. The child is often able to give reinforcement and feedback about the parent's effectiveness in meeting needs. The parent is also helped to determine when a child's demands are excessive or when he, the parent, can make demands. After a bedtime story and a kiss, for example, it is perfectly all right to expect a child to go to sleep. A four-year-old child, in a family setting, does not need a parent to stay with him while he falls asleep. When a parent likes to have the living room picked up in the evening, he has every right to ask a child to pick up his toys or insist that he at least participate in this task.

To participate successfully in a nurturing relationship, a person must have need satisfaction from a source or sources other than the nurturing partner. In other words, a person must feel safe and know there will be a continuous supply of love and respect available with minimal effort on his part. Given this, an individual is free to devote time and attention to the person in need of nurturing. The therapist must be aware of this requirement, since it may be necessary to give additional fulfillment as a parent learns to take on the nurturing role. The parent must also be helped to find some way of securing adequate need satisfaction in the community. Participation in a parents' discussion group may help him to find ways of altering his life situation so that he receives support for his role as a parent.

One difficulty that may occur in the area of nurturing is overinvolvement with the nurturing partner. Norm, for example, who taught fourth grade in a ghetto school, spent at least seventy-two hours a week at the school. He was involved in the breakfast program, after-school care projects, and the Saturday tutorial-recreation service as well as teaching his class every day. When he was not at school, he was worrying about the children. In order to help Norm with this problem, the therapist suggested he work for two hours in a nursing home not far from the treatment center. Shortly after beginning the job, Norm started to work more than two hours and developed the same intense relationship with the residents that he had had with his students. The therapist did not suggest that Norm return to his school part-time because he had assured her his involvement was only due to the students having so many and unique needs. Seeing the same pattern occur in a different setting, Norm was more able to recognize his difficulty with nurturing relationships. Using his daily experiences in the nursing home, Norm and the therapist talked about his ideas, feelings, and values relative to the nurturing process. He was helped to see that his desire "to save the world" was, to some extent, unrealistic, and ultimately detrimental to the need satisfaction of himself and others. Ways of decreasing involvement were discussed and tried.

Giving up a nurturing relationship is difficult for some people. They essentially want to hang on to the partner even after he no longer needs nurturing. Betty, a private duty nurse, became depressed and anxious after finishing each assignment. She only worked periodically, since she was also a participant in a handcrafted gift store cooperative. After considerable discussion Betty realized that, first, she strongly suspected "her" patients were not going to get adequate care after she left the case, and that, second, caring for people was more important to her than being a craftsman. This latter idea was difficult for Betty to accept. The other store cooperative members, of whom she was very fond, thought nursing was "passing out bed pans and taking temperatures." Betty went back to nursing full time on the night shift. This enabled her to allay her fear that patients were not being cared for properly and still spend time with her friends. She soon found it much easier to move out of a nurturing relationship.

Summary

Teaching in the area of intimacy is rather indirect for the therapist. It is helping the patient to be "out there" engaging with others. This is disturbing to some therapists. They may feel a sense of loss as the patient becomes more distant from them. These are common feelings a therapist accepts and learns to live with. They arise because the therapist likes the patient, and treatment could not occur without that liking. The negative feelings are usually counterbalanced by joy that the patient is able to participate in shared intimate relations with others.

SUGGESTED READING

Frye, V., and Peter, M. *Therapeutic Recreation.* Harrisburg, Pa.: The Stackpole Company, 1972.

Hoppock, Robert. *Occupational Information.* New York: McGraw-Hill Book Company, 1967.

Thompson, Nellie. *The Role of the Workshop in Rehabilitation.* Washington, D.C.: U.S. Department of Health, Education and Welfare, 1968.

U.S. Department of Health, Education, and Welfare. *Workshops for the Disabled.* Washington, D.C.: Office of Vocational Rehabilitation, 1965.

CHAPTER 10

DEVELOPMENT OF FACETS
OF THE PRIVATE SELF

Facets of the private self—cognitive system, needs, emotions, and values—are interdependent. For example, a person may not be able to satisfy his need for mastery because he thinks he is totally inept. Another person may not be able to express anger because he believes it is wrong to do so. Because of this interdependence, treatment in the area of the private self usually takes all facets into consideration collectively. A patient is helped to look at typical faulty behavior patterns and discover what facets of the private self account for these ineffective ways of behaving. He is then assisted in changing these facets if he so desires. Although usually dealt with collectively in the actual treatment situation, the first section of this chapter is devoted to discussion of each individual facet of the private self.

DEVELOPMENT OF ISOLATED FACETS OF THE PRIVATE SELF

Cognitive System

Some patients do not know enough about the world around them to interact in that world. As mentioned in previous chapters, some patients, for example, know very little about their neighborhood, how to interact with large institutions, what to wear to a job interview, how to shop for groceries, and so forth. Patients are helped to gain information by someone explaining what they need to know or through the experience of interacting in the unfamiliar situation or both. This process was examined in some detail in previous chapters and will not be discussed further here.

One difficulty in the area of cognitive system is inaccurate ideas about oneself or other people. These ideas may be conscious or unconscious.

Ideas about oneself and others are gained through experience, and what other people, who are important to the individual, have indicated was true. For example, Mike thinks he is a good basketball player because he frequently gets the ball into the basket and because his coach has him play as much as possible in each game. Once a person gets an idea about himself or others, he tends to hold on to that idea. Someone who believes, for example, that other people are not to be trusted may maintain that belief regardless of whether he is with people who are trustworthy or with those who are not. Similarly, someone who sees himself as a failure manages to fail in many different circumstances.

Although people sometimes change deeply ingrained ideas about themselves or others through casual interaction in unplanned situations, patients rarely seem to have this capacity. Several steps are usually necessary to bring about a change in faulty ideas about the self and others. First, the patient is helped to become aware of an idea if it is not conscious. This is done by suggesting various ideas to the patient. Suggestions are made based on what the therapist thinks the patient believes about himself or others. The patient may reject several ideas before he finds one that seems to be what he really thinks. The idea is then discussed. Is it true or false? Is this idea commonly held by others? This process is sometimes referred to as *reality testing*. An idea previously unconscious or generally kept secret by the individual is exposed to the light of day. It is examined to help the patient decide whether, in the present circumstances, this is a valid, useful idea.

This examination, however, may not be sufficient in and of itself for a person to give up an invalid idea. He may have to experiment in a variety of situations before he is able to accept a more valid idea. To illustrate, Erik rarely participated in any group discussion; he sat in the corner, observant, but silent. Erik's difficulty became the focus of the group. When questioned about his silence, Erik said he was shy. The group felt this was too vague to be of any use and began to suggest ideas Erik might have about himself or the group. After rejecting several suggestions, Erik agreed that he believed no one could possibly be interested in his opinions. The majority of the group said that as far as they were concerned this was not true; they would very much like to hear his opinions. Reassurance was not sufficient to change Erik's idea about other people, but it did, with the support of the group, enable Erik to begin occasionally to express his opinion in the group. As is true with most patients who have faulty ideas about themselves or other people, Erik needed practice in acting in a way that was contrary to his deeply rooted ideas. For example, Erik at first expressed his opinions in such a way that no one could really understand what he was trying to say. Rather than only half listening, the group took time out to help Erik state his opinions more clearly. Later it was necessary for the group to help Erik state his opinion as his own. Erik had a tendency to begin each statement with such expressions as, "Most people think . . ." or "In general one could say. . . ." It took considerable group encouragement for Erik to be able to begin a statement of opinion with "I think. . . ." As time went on, group members urged Erik to express his opinion in situations other than the group. Erik found that, indeed, in many situations people were quite willing to listen to what he had to say. Slowly Erik's idea about other people changed.

Some patients are unaware of what they are doing and the effect of their behavior on other people. They believe they are behaving in one way although they are actually doing something entirely different. They are either confused about the response they get from the other person, interpret the response incorrectly, or pay no attention to how the other person is responding. Richard, for example, actually thought he was being supportive when he quizzed another patient as if the patient were on the witness stand. Nicole was totally unaware that people thought her frequent pleas for help sounded much more like demands. A patient with difficulty in this area needs someone to provide massive doses of feedback. This seems to be most effective immediately after the behavior occurs. Lack of knowledge about one's own behavior and response to that behavior is identified by comparing the patient's behavior to what appears to be called for in the situation. Asking the patient to talk about what he thought he was doing and asking the other participant in the interaction to talk about how he interpreted the patient's behavior serves as the beginning point for change. The interchange is studied by persons who are not immediately involved. They provide feedback to the patient regarding the relationship between what he said he was doing and what he appeared to be doing and the validity of the other participant's interpretation. The point here is not to help a patient immediately alter his behavior. Rather, it is to assist him in identifying what he is doing and the effect of his behavior on others. The therapist and other group members help the patient become "self-conscious" about his behavior—to know, essentially, "What am I doing now?" The patient is assisted in learning how to study the effects of his actions. When there is adequate feedback, reinforcement, and opportunity for trial-and-error learning, repeated requests to talk about one's own behavior and the response of others helps a patient gain knowledge about his behavior and the reactions of others. Learning is enhanced if the patient is encouraged to talk about interactions that are effective as well as about those that are ineffective.

Assisting a patient to understand his assets and limitations is similar to treatment of other problems in the cognitive area. A person who does not know what he is and is not able to do tends to think either that he can do far more than he is able or far less. Patients who are truly inadequate in many aspects of their functioning, and know this is true, have no difficulty in this area. The ideal way of helping patients understand their assets and limitations is to place them in situations where they are able to test their skills and abilities. A patient who believes he has no problems relative to work, for example, may be placed in a work situation. The patient can then experience what he is and is not able to do. When necessary, the therapist or work supervisor provides feedback—telling the patient what he has done well and what he has done poorly. Some patients make excuses for poor performance. They blame someone or something else in the situation for their poor performance. The therapist continues to describe what is occurring as accurately as possible. The idea that it is perfectly all right to recognize both assets and limitations is communicated to the patient.

Needs

Patients who have difficulty recognizing their needs experience dissatisfaction without having any idea of what is causing the dissatisfaction. One way of helping such patients is to talk to them about needs. This is often done through completion of the Activity Configuration discussed in Chapter 6. The therapist and patient attempt to identify what needs the patient is not satisfying. They discuss various ways the patient could satisfy unmet needs. The patient is encouraged to try one or several of the discussed ideas. The consequence of this trial action is examined at a later date to determine if the activity was or was not need satisfying. Other activities are tried if the initial activities were not need gratifying.

The treatment process is not, however, always so simple as described above. Some patients cannot recognize a need even when their behavior indicates a high degree of need deprivation. In this case, the therapist attempts to interpret the patient's nonverbal behavior. What need does the patient *seem* to be experiencing at the present time? The therapist suggests to the patient the need she thinks he is experiencing. If the patient rejects the suggested need, another need is offered for consideration. This process is similar to the process described for helping a person identify the ideas he has about himself and others. Sometimes, when a patient cannot identify a need, the therapist may provide satisfaction of the need she believes the patient is experiencing. A patient, for example, may appear to be troubled and confused by the fairly unstructured nature of the treatment setting. The therapist makes out a detailed schedule for the patient to follow. If the patient appears to be more comfortable after the therapist has provided need satisfaction, they can be fairly certain they have identified the patient's need correctly. In addition, a patient may be encouraged to move in and out of a need-satisfying situation. He is then in a position to experience what satisfaction and deprivation of that need feel like. Using the above example to illustrate, the patient may be provided with a schedule only every other day. The therapist helps the patient identify the difference between how he feels when he has a schedule and when he does not have a schedule.

After a patient has learned to identify needs, it is sometimes necessary to help him learn how to satisfy his needs. Initially, the therapist may gratify the patient's needs. When the patient is ready to learn to satisfy a need himself, however, the therapist limits her need satisfaction to some extent. Mild deprivation tends to facilitate learning. Teaching a patient how to satisfy needs will vary according to the specific problems the patient is having in satisfying a need. Thus, the following discussion is not inclusive of everything that might be done to help a patient.

Physiological Needs. Teaching activities of daily living and work habits is one way of assisting a patient to satisfy physiological needs. When a patient is unable to work, he may need to learn how to apply for welfare money and how to manage in the bureaucratic welfare system. The area of recreation may also require exploration, in order for the patient to maintain an optimal level of sensory stimuli and motor activity. Many patients have difficulty satisfying their sexual needs. At times, it is useful for a patient to explore ideas, emotions, and values that appear to be interfering with satisfaction of his sexual needs. This may be done on a one-to-one basis with the therapist or in a group situation. Sometimes a person is unable to satisfy his sexual needs because of difficulties in the area of intimacy. When this is the case, the therapist helps the patient to develop skill in this area. Finally, the patient may lack knowledge or be misinformed about sexual matters. If the therapist does not feel she is able to provide adequate explanation, she helps the patient to find someone who is able to do so.

Safety Needs. There seem to be three common problems in meeting the need to be in a living situation that is perceived as safe. The patient may actually live in a physically unsafe neighborhood. The rate of street crime and household robbery may, for example, be quite high. Ideally, the therapist helps the patient find a more safe place to live. However, this is not always possible. The therapist then helps the patient learn to take reasonable precautions, such as carrying only a small amount of money, walking on the curb side of the sidewalk, taking a longer but more well-traveled route to one's destination, having a secure lock for one's door, being acutely aware of the other people on the street, not arguing with a mugger, and the like. The patient may also be helped to locate someone else in his apartment building or nearby who can accompany him on at least some of his trips out into the community.

Another problem in meeting safety needs has to do with living in a psychologically unsafe environment. A patient's home situation may, for example, be one in which responses from others are not predictable and most decisions are made in an arbitrary fashion. The patient may be helped to alter his home situation by asking family members to change their behavior. The patient explains why he feels change is needed and provides reinforcement for appropriate change. This is often a difficult task, and patients need considerable support in bringing about change in a family situation. Another way of making the home environment more safe for the patient is for a staff member to intervene. The problem with this method is that the patient is not an active participant in satisfying his own safety needs. He is not learning how to gratify this need through his own actions. When possible, family activities therapy is a better alternative. The patient is urged to take an active role in identifying ways in which family members act that cause him to feel unsafe. The ideas, needs, emotions, and values leading to need-depriving patterns of behavior are explored and, if possible, identified and examined. The patient and other family members are encouraged to try other types of behavior.

When the family is not able to participate in family therapy and the patient is not able to bring about change through his own efforts, the patient may attempt to learn to tolerate the situation. There are two approaches that may make this possible. One is to help the patient realize what is occurring in his family situation—to know when the situation is and is not gratifying his need for safety. Through understanding of the situation and his own responses, the patient is often able to withdraw psychologically and delay gratification of his need for safety. In other words, the patient is helped to identify what is occurring in family interactions, to learn that this is what is causing him to feel confused and anxious, and to be able to say, "I am not going to pay any attention, I'm not going to let this bother me." The other factor that can help the patient tolerate a relatively unsafe home environment is to assist him in finding a group of other people who allow him to meet his safety needs. The patient is given help in finding and interacting with friends, co-workers, work supervisors, and the like who appreciate the importance of meeting safety needs. These are the type of people, for example, who clearly communicate what is expected and desirable behavior and who allow the patient to influence their actions.

When the patient cannot tolerate continued lack of gratification of his safety needs in the home situation, he may be helped to move out of the home. Such a move is usually traumatic for both the patient and his family; considerable support is required. The patient may need help in finding a place to live. He may also have to learn some activities of daily living that were not required of him in his home situation. If the patient is going to be living with a group of other people, he may need to acquire additional skills in interpersonal relations.

Some patients are unable to meet their safety needs because they do not know enough about common situations. They may, for example, know little about their neighborhood, where to shop, and how to use public transportation. Or they may not be able to interpret other people's responses. Thus, they do not know what is expected of them or what other people are likely to do. Patients with this type of difficulty have often just recently moved into the community from a very dissimilar type of community. Others, however, have simply not learned to manage ordinary life situations. These patients are helped by being assisted to learn required activities of daily living and group-interaction skills. They are given the opportunity to interact in a variety of different situations both in the treatment center and in the wider community. Adequate and consistent feedback is important.

Love and Belonging Needs. Patients who have difficulty meeting their need for love and belonging usually have limitations in the area of intimacy and group-interaction skill. Helping a patient develop skill in these areas has been discussed previously (see pages 163–169), so a description of the process will not be repeated here. One common problem with patients who have difficulty satisfying love and belonging needs is that they attempt to satisfy these needs in the wrong situations. They cannot differentiate between situations where one is likely to have love and belonging needs met and situations where this is unlikely to occur. As a result, their efforts to satisfy these needs often meet with failure. These patients need help in learning to interpret situations. For example, a student is probably not going to get his need for belonging satisfied by attending classes in large lecture halls. However, this need may be satisfied by participating in a small student organization.

Sometimes patients, in attempting to understand the need for love and belonging, are confused when it is identified as the need to be accepted for oneself rather than acceptance for what one has done or is doing. They see this as meaning that they do not have to act in any particular way to be accepted; they should just be able to demand acceptance and it will automatically be given. This misconception must be clarified for the patient. He is helped to realize that there are certain minimal standards of behavior required for acceptance in most situations. And love is rarely offered without something being given in return. It is only in relationships such as those between parent and young child or therapist and patient that love is given unconditionally.

Mastery Needs. The first step in helping a patient learn to satisfy his need for mastery involves identification of the patient's interests, temperament, and assets and limitations. The patient is encouraged to think about activities he might enjoy which would offer him some degree of challenge. The therapist suggests activities that are not so easy for the patient as to require little effort on his part or so difficult that he will become discouraged. Often the patient tries several different activities before he is able to determine the kind of activity that will meet his need for mastery. As in the area of recreation, the activities with which the patient experiments should be the kinds of activities he will be able to pursue in his home community.

Sometimes patients have difficulty meeting their need for mastery because they have the idea they cannot do anything well or they fear failure or both. These patients are helped initially to identify these often unconscious ideas and emotions. While examining these facets of the self within the context of the present situation, a patient is helped to understand that, although there may always be some things he will not be able to master, there are aspects of himself and the environment that he can master. A patient may be assisted in altering his ideas and emotional responses by encouraging him to participate in a graduated series of enjoyable activities which are increasingly challenging to him. These graduated activities are carefully selected by the patient and therapist so that the patient is likely to have a successful experience. The adjective *likely* should be emphasized: If success is assured, the activity will not be challenging. Activities that are not to some degree challenging do not satisfy the need for mastery. Failure is always possible in any activity undertaken for the sake of meeting mastery needs. A patient who fears failure often must experience failure in order to gain control over this emotional response. Through such experience the patient comes to see that the consequences of failure are rarely catastrophic; neither he nor the world falls apart. The patient, of course, will require considerable initial support. He is helped to accept failure and not flee the situation, blame failure on others, or deny that he failed. Accepting failure and determining what to do about it brings the patient a long way toward meeting his mastery needs.

Esteem Needs. What can the patient do or learn to do that will enable him to receive respect from other people? Who are these other people? These are the two major questions that guide the teaching-learning process in helping a patient satisfy esteem needs. Sometimes a patient wants respect from people who have too high or unacceptable expectations. He cannot gain their respect because he is unable or unwilling to meet their expectations. An example would be the parents who want their daughter to go to college and prepare for one of the professions. The daughter is not academically inclined, and, besides, she wants to become a policewoman. The patient is helped first to sort out the situation: "Who do I want respect from? Can I meet the expectations of these people? Do I want to meet these expectations?" Once these questions are answered, the patient is in a position to select a course of action. He can try to get people who are important to him to change their expectations. He can decide to meet the expectations even though they are somewhat different from what he would like to do. He can decide that he either cannot or will not meet the expectations. The therapist assists the patient, if necessary, in carrying out these decisions.

When the latter choice is made, the patient often has to decrease his emotional investment in people to whom he had looked for satisfaction of his esteem needs. He must find other people to satisfy these needs. These must be people who respect a person for doing the type of thing the patient wants to do. For example, David, who wants to be a barber, usually interacts with people who believe barbering is not a very worthy occupation. It was necessary for the therapist and other members of his work discussion group to fulfill David's esteem needs until he was able to have these needs met by the instructors and students at barber school.

Patients unable to satisfy esteem needs in a work situation are helped to find other ways of satisfying these needs. The process of doing this is similar to that discussed with regard to treatment in the area of recreation. However, rather than asking, "Is this the kind of activity that will give me a sense of relaxation and enjoyment?", the patient experiments with various activities to determine whether they fulfill his esteem needs. Making things that are appreciated by or useful to others and participating in community organizations are fairly common ways of satisfying esteem needs.

Perhaps the most difficult patients to help in this area are those who are able to make only a marginal adjustment to community living. They have few skills that enable them to fulfill esteem needs. It takes a great deal of ingenuity and time to find some place in the community where these patients can get at least some need satisfaction. A sheltered workshop might be suitable if there is one in the community. The patient may be able to do volunteer work that involves fairly simple tasks. Sometimes a small shopkeeper is willing to hire the patient for a few hours each day. There usually is a place for the patient, if only the place can be found.

Self-actualization Needs. People who have difficulty meeting their need for self-actualization sometimes have guilt feelings about satisfying this need. They feel that the time they would be spending in meeting this need should be devoted to other things. "I should spend the time with my family" or "I have too many responsibilities at work" are common responses to an inquiry about self-actualization needs. The individual has set priorities in such a manner that meeting self-actualization needs comes last. If necessary, a patient is assisted in identifying his priorities. He must know what his priorities are before he is able to decide whether or not this is a satisfactory way to order his life. The patient is encouraged to examine his weekly activities to determine whether the time allotted for each activity is the amount of time he needs or wants to spend in that activity. Further, the patient is helped to understand that meeting self-actualization needs is not necessarily selfish or detrimental to the need satisfaction of others. Some patients do not have any idea about what sort of activities will satisfy their need for self-actualization. Even after deciding they want to devote time to fulfilling this need, they do not know what to do. In this case the therapist encourages the patient to try a variety of different activities, in order to test whether the activity gratifies his self-actualization need. This may take some time, because the patient must find a way to express his own special sense of self—a difficult task for many people.

One other area of concern for the therapist is to help patients delay satisfaction or learn to live with a moderate amount of need deprivation. This is done by very slowly diminishing satisfaction of a need while ensuring that the patient's need is met ultimately either in the specific treatment situation or in other situations. For example, in helping Ken delay satisfaction of his need for esteem, the therapist originally complimented him for successful completion of every step of an activity. Recognition of work well done was slowly decreased; only completion of major steps resulted in attention. Finally, the therapist gave approval only after successful completion of an entire activity. Another example may be useful: To help Jill tolerate the deprivation of her need for mastery that she experienced at work, the therapist assisted her in making arrangements to participate in a community center arts-and-crafts program. The therapist also helps patients to anticipate need-depriving events. She gives patients suggestions about regulating their life, if possible, so that they receive need gratification from other sources while they are going through a need-depriving experience. It may be suggested, for example, that a patient not take on additional responsibilities at work and move into a new apartment at the same time, or if a close companion is going away for a week, to plan ahead to visit with friends several evenings that week.

Emotions

Learning in the area of emotional expression can take place only in a treatment center where there is a high positive value placed on adequate emotional expression. As previously defined, adequate emotional expression is expression that is sufficient to inhibit the formation of an uncomfortable amount of internal tension and sufficiently controlled so as not to interfere with current or future need fulfillment. Excessive expression of emotion is allowed and even encouraged if such expression leads to learning adequate emotional expression. The only rule relative to excessive expression of emotion is usually that patients are not allowed to injure another person or destroy property. Participants in a treatment center occasionally get carried away with the need to express emotion. Inadvertently, a norm develops that implies that excessive emotional expression is good in and of itself. The problem with this norm is that excessive emotional expression is not acceptable in many sectors of the wider community. A patient who has learned excessive rather than adequate emotional expression is often confused about and unprepared to conform to the norms of the wider community.

There seem to be two types of difficulty with emotional expression: It is either too controlled or too excessive. Some patients, however, have difficulty in both areas. The situation determines how they express emotions. Patients who are too controlled in emotional expression sometimes seem to be unaware of the emotions they are experiencing. They either cannot label the emotion or they mislabel it, as, for example, in the case of a patient who says he is depressed when his behavior strongly suggests he is angry. In attempting to help this type of patient, the therapist may go through the process of suggesting possible emotions the patient may be experiencing. This is similar to the process of helping a patient identify his needs.

Suggestions are made tentatively allowing the patient to try to get at or to the level of his feelings. No pressure is applied; the patient is encouraged to reject any suggestions that do not seem to apply to his emotional state. Another way of helping the patient is to urge him to express what he feels. There is no attempt to label the emotion; that can wait until later. The patient is simply urged to say what he is thinking and to act out how he feels. He usually needs considerable support to be able to do this. The process of shaping may be of assistance. If this learning technique is used, any expression of emotion is reinforced until the patient is able to express his emotions. Patients who are unable to express their emotions often have ideas and values that prohibit display of emotions. Ideas vary from, "Any expression of negative feelings can actually cause physical harm to another person," to, "Only weak and 'feminine' people express positive emotions." A high negative value is placed on all of these ideas. A patient is helped to discover his ideas and values related to emotional expression. When necessary, this is, again, done through suggesting possible values and ideas for the patient's consideration. The patient is urged to talk about his ideas and values and to test whether, in his present circumstances, these ideas and values are reasonable and useful. Feedback is an important element in this process.

Other factors that facilitate the learning of adequate emotional expression are opportunities for trial-and-error experimentation, models for imitation, and role playing. Patients are encouraged to try various ways of expressing their emotions both in the more structured circumstances of an activities therapy group and in casual interactions in the treatment center. The patient is given feedback. But the atmosphere of the treatment center is sufficiently free so that the consequence of somewhat bizarre expression is not as negative as it would be in the wider community. Trial expression is encouraged and accepted for what it is: an attempt to learn. Staff members often serve as the primary models for imitation. Thus, it is important for staff members to be open in their expression of both positive and negative emotions. Affection for other staff members is freely demonstrated, and disagreements are openly discussed. Role playing offers an additional opportunity for experimentation and imitation. Incidents for role playing may be taken from an event that has recently occurred in the group or from a situation in which one of the group members was involved in the treatment center or wider community. The patient may take his own role in order to attempt to express his emotions more adequately. Or another group member, more skilled in emotional expression, may take the role of the patient to demonstrate one way of expressing a particular emotion. Reinforcement and feedback are freely given.

Because the adequate expression of emotions is often easier in the accepting atmosphere of the treatment center than in the community, patients frequently need help in learning to express their emotions in settings other than the treatment center. A patient needs an opportunity to experiment with emotional expression in the community and to discuss this experimentation with other patients and staff members. In this discussion, the patient is able to report back on his efforts and to receive advice and support from the group.

The above-suggested ways of helping patients who are too controlled in their display of emotions may also be used to help patients who are too excessive in their display of emotions. However, another factor may be involved in the excessive display of emotions. A patient sometimes expresses emotions in one situation that actually developed through interaction in another or several other situations. Rather than expressing the emotion at the time and place the emotion was aroused, the patient "saved" expression for a later time. The storing up of emotional expression often increases the intensity of the emotion. Some small incident in a later situation may set off or trigger expression of previously stored emotion. Such expression is often explosive. It comes as somewhat of a surprise to participants in the later situation, because the emotional expression seems unrelated to the events that have just taken place. The first step in helping a patient who displaces emotional expression from one situation to another is to explore the present situation and the patient's ideas about the situation. An attempt is made to identify what there is in the present situation that is similar to past situations in which the patient could not express negative emotions. This usually takes considerable time and discussion. Explosive emotional expression may have to occur several times before the right relationship is found. For example, Leo became extremely angry at three different group members and the therapist over a period of several days. The group looked at what each of these persons was actually doing at the time Leo became angry and how Leo had perceived these actions. The common element turned out to be that either the group members had talked positively about leaving the treatment center or Leo had thought this was how they were talking. Further discussion revealed that Leo's primary therapist and people in the sheltered workshop were urging Leo to begin making plans to leave the center. Leo had been unable to express his fears about leaving or to ask for the help he felt he needed. He was angry about these demands but had been unable to express his anger. It was also discovered that this had been a typical pattern of behavior for Leo prior to coming to the treatment center.

When an individual displaces emotional expression from one situation to another, the difficulty is sometimes not inadequate emotional expression. Rather, the problem may be difficulty in altering situations that lead to the arousal of intense emotions. Anger and fear are common responses to being placed in a position of not knowing how to gain at least some control over the situation. Thus the teaching-learning process is directed toward helping the patient deal with certain types of situations as opposed to focusing on emotional expression. Returning to the example above, Leo had to learn how to tell people he could not meet their demands at this time and that he needed extra help if he was going to meet these demands in the future. Leo practiced doing this in his daily living group, and group members gave him considerable support in expressing these ideas to the people at the sheltered workshop.

Vigorous activities, such as pounding, scrubbing a floor, or active sports, are sometimes suggested for patients who have problems with anger. These activities may be suggested to patients who do not seem to know they are angry. The patient and therapist then examine how the patient performed the activity and his feelings during participation in the activity. It is sometimes easier for a patient to recognize his anger when he sees it manifested in his actions. Other patients seem to need to learn how to engage in vigorous activities before they are able to begin focusing on their own angry feelings. Vigorous activities may also be suggested to patients who know they are angry, but who are having difficulty controlling expression of their anger. Active participation in vigorous activities seems temporarily to "drain off" excessive anger. Expending considerable energy appears to diminish the intensity of anger for a period of time. Given temporary relief, the patient is often more able to examine his feelings of anger and to find out what he needs to learn in order to avoid becoming so angry. Vigorous activities are only one part of the process of helping patients deal with anger. They cannot, in and of themselves, lead to adequate emotional expression.

Values

Values are a touchy subject for many people. Thinking about values varies from one extreme—"There is only one right system of values"—to the other extreme—"No one has the right to say that one system of values is better than any other system." Activities therapists are not concerned with imposing a value system, but neither do they ignore the area of values. Patients are helped to become aware of their values and to discover if, in fact, these are the values they wish to have. The more aware a person is of his values, the better he is able to determine whether these are values that will allow him to meet his needs without interfering with the need satisfaction of others.

The atmosphere of the treatment center is important in assisting patients to identify and, if desirable, to change values. Ideally, participants in the treatment center are, collectively, self-conscious about the values that determine the norms of the center. The collective values of the center are frequently discussed to find out whether they are, in fact, contributing to the teaching-learning process that is supposed to be taking place in the center. There is a conscious effort to alter collective values detrimental to learning. Such an atmosphere provides a model for identification and change of personal values.

Patients are assisted to look at their values as these values are reflected in their actions. A patient who is consistently late for all appointments, for example, is helped to identify the value he places on "lateness" and "being on time." The value identified may be consistent with the patient's actions, or it may be quite the opposite. The patient and therapist attempt to determine if the stated value is more truly reflective of the patient's beliefs or if the patient's actions are closer to what the patient actually believes. To use the above example, the patient who is always late for appointments may say that being late is bad; he really tries to be on time but something always happens. This may be true: The patient thinks it is wrong to be late. Other factors such as not being able to organize himself sufficiently to be on time, or not liking the people he is supposed to see at an appointed time, may contribute to his lateness. On the other hand, the patient may only be paying lip service to the idea that it is good to be on time. Actually, being late is of little concern to him; he will get somewhere when he gets there.

After identifying a value, the patient must decide if he wants to make any changes. He has several options: no, he does not want to alter the value because he does not think it in any way diminishes his need satisfaction or the need satisfaction of other people; no, he wants to keep the value but he does not want to learn to live up to the value; or, yes, he wants to change the value. In the case of ambivalence, assigning both a negative and positive value to an idea, event, person, and so forth, the patient must decide which value is more need fulfilling for him. The therapist and fellow group members help the patient reach a decision about value change by talking about both the likely negative and likely positive consequences of making a change or not making a change.

One way in which values are acquired is through experience. A person comes to place a high positive value on persons, events, and ideas that contribute to need satisfaction. High negative values are assigned to persons, events, and ideas that lead to need deprivation. Using this idea about how values are acquired, the therapist designs learning experiences that will help a patient act as if he held the desired value. Situations are designed so that the patient receives need satisfaction as a result of acting in accordance with the new value. For example, Carl wanted to alter his negative value toward manual labor of any kind. Therefore, he was strongly encouraged to get heavily involved in the weekly general cleaning session at the day treatment center and to spend three hours each day working at a local gas station. Carl was given much attention and praise for his work. He was also given ample opportunity to talk about his feelings and his work experiences. Eventually Carl came to take pride in his work. He began to experience pleasure in a job well done. This same method is used when a patient wants to learn how to act in accordance with a value he already holds. Thus, for example, the patient who believes it is a good thing to be able to dress nicely, even with limited funds, is helped to learn something about budgeting, clothes repair and alteration, where to shop, and so on.

Another way an individual acquires values is to take on the values of other people who are seen as need fulfilling. He accepts the values of these other people because he thinks this will contribute to his general state of need satisfaction. This method of acquiring values is also used in the treatment situation. For example, Nina wanted to limit her family to one child. However, this course of action would probably lead to the loss of several friends and alienation from both her own and her husband's relatives. Nina was helped to join and participate in the work of a chapter of the Planned Parenthood Association. Nina was able to satisfy many of her needs for belonging and esteem through involvement with the Association. In this situation, Nina's high regard for family planning led to need fulfillment. Another patient, Milt, knew he would no longer be able to work at a paying job. He was highly ambivalent about retiring,

but did agree to join a senior citizens' organization, "just to try it out."
Milt found participation in the activities of the organization very enjoyable. He began to see retirement as not being so bad after all.

Summary

This section has discussed treatment in the area of the private self. Each facet of the overall pattern was discussed separately so that the reader might sense some of the specifics involved in the teaching-learning process. We now turn to an examination of the pattern as a whole. Because of the interdependence of facets of the private self, difficulties in this area are often altered by focusing on all of the facets collectively. The following section discusses an activities group designed primarily to effect change in the private self.

COLLECTIVE DEVELOPMENT

An activities therapy group specially designed to develop aspects of the private self may be made up of a heterogeneous or homogeneous group of patients or a family. In a heterogeneous group, the only characteristic shared by all the patients is some difficulty in facets of the private self. In a homogeneous group, the patients share additional characteristics. The group, for example, may be made up only of women or only of men. Members may all have a common medical diagnosis, such as drug addiction or adolescent adjustment reaction. A family activities therapy group is usually made up of all the members of an immediate family over the age of six or seven. Relations who are closely involved with the family may also participate. One family member may have been designated as the patient, or the family as a whole may have sought help with their difficulties in interacting. Family activities therapy usually takes place in a treatment center, making use of activities facilities used by patients during the day. However, some family activities therapy may take place in the family home. This often allows younger children to be involved in the treatment process. The family's usual evening activities are then used as the vehicle for treatment.

The role of the therapist in a group concerned primarily with development of the private self is not significantly different from that of other group members. Therefore, her role is not singled out in the discussion that follows. All group members, including the therapist, play an active role in helping individuals gain better self-understanding and to alter, if desired, aspects of the self. The planning and execution of group tasks is the vehicle for learning. Almost any task that can be shared in some way is suitable. However, the task must be such that it can remain secondary. Interruptions must be possible, and there must be no scheduled time for completion. The task may have an end product, such as a large doll house, or it may have no visible end product, such as reading poetry or going swimming. The format of the group usually is to work at the task, to interrupt the task to facilitate learning, to return to the task, and so on. There is usually a period set aside at the end of each group meeting for general discussion.

The learning process within the group involves consideration repetition of five basic steps: (1) What is going on here? (2) Exploration, (3) What needs to be changed? (4) Learning, and (5) Follow-up.

What Is Going on Here?

Some people refer to this step as *encounter* or *confrontation*. However, these words have a negative connotation for some people. There is often the feeling of attacking or putting someone "on the spot." "What is going on here" refers to some group member observing an event in the group or experiencing some feeling or idea and calling the group's attention to this phenomenon. The phenomenon may be negative, such as one patient ignoring another patient's request for help, or a sudden feeling of anxiety. It may be more neutral, such as one patient seemingly wandering aimlessly around the room while everyone else is working. Or it may be positive, such as a patient who always deferred to the therapist as the authority suddenly arguing with the therapist, or another patient who becomes aware that he really feels good today in this group meeting.

Negative phenomena are called to the group's attention to help the person or persons involved discover what is going on. More neutral phenomena are identified to determine whether there is a problem. For example, someone may be wandering around the room because he is bored. That is a problem. On the other hand, he may just need at the time to be with another person. He is wandering around to feel out whether someone would not mind being interrupted for a few minutes. Positive phenomena are made note of, both to share delight in new learning or another person's good feelings and, if considered important, to find out how this was brought about.

This step simply involves stopping whatever is going on in the group by saying something like,"I want to look at what's happening," or, "I suddenly thought of something I want to share." Questions such as "What do you think you are doing?" or "Why did you do that?" are avoided. Calling the group's attention to something is done gently, without suggesting that a member has done something wrong. It is a norm of this group to give attention to anyone who takes the first step in the learning process.

Exploration

Exploration is essentially a verbal process. It is, first, an examination of the actual situation. When two or more people are involved in an event, they are each asked to describe what was happening: not how they felt or the reason for their behavior but simply, "What were you doing and what were the other people doing?" For example, "I (Hugo) said such and such, and Margaret walked out of the room," not, "I was trying to get Margaret to agree with me." Other, uninvolved group members provide feedback about what they saw and the sequence of events. The group as a whole discusses the event until there is some sort of general agreement about what actually happened. This helps the group obtain a common point of reference and helps the involved members acquire a sense of what they were actually doing.

Next, each involved patient is urged to talk about what he thought was happening, what ideas about himself were brought to mind, his emotional responses, the needs he was experiencing, and the values he places on all these factors in the situation. For example, Margaret, a patient with some experience in the group, might say, "I thought Hugo was telling me what to do and that made me feel like a little girl. I don't know what emotion I was feeling. And I do not like to be told what to do or to feel like a little girl. I walked out of the room because I felt badly and couldn't think of anything else to do."

The group helps the patient check whether his perception of the event was relatively accurate. Hugo says he was trying to get Margaret to agree with him; Margaret says differently. The group, after some discussion, agrees with Margaret. Hugo was coming across very strongly: His request sounded like a demand. Margaret's perception was accurate.

Next, the group tries to help the patient identify ideas about himself and the situation, emotions, needs, and values that he is unable to talk about or appears to be talking about inaccurately. This is done by trying to "read" the patient's nonverbal behavior: his facial expressions, body posture, actions, and so forth. Also, knowing something about the event, group members are able to draw on their past experience in similar situations: how they had felt, what emotions had been aroused, what needs had not been satisfied, and so forth. Individual members in the group give feedback to the patient about what they felt the patient was experiencing. With this individualized feedback the patient gains several suggestions about possible needs, ideas, emotions, and values of which he seems to be unaware. The patient is given an opportunity to compare internal states with suggestions about what these states might be. He may find that one of the suggestions is accurate; it identifies one aspect of his internal experience; it seems to fit. At other times a patient may reject all suggestions: No, that was not what he was thinking or feeling. Pressure is never placed on the patient to accept a suggestion even when many group members give the same feedback. It is his *private* existence that is being explored. He has the right to accept or reject other people's ideas about his needs and values. If the pattern of internal experiences and behavior is typical of the patient, it will occur again in the group setting. Next time, perhaps, the patient will be better able to talk about himself and about what is happening with him.

To return to our earlier example, Margaret did not mention any needs and did not know what emotions she was experiencing. In addition, several group members raised the question of whether Margaret really placed a negative value on the idea that she was like a little girl. Some group members felt that Margaret was experiencing a strong need for love, others that she wanted her esteem needs met. Fear, anger, and hatred were suggested as possible emotions. When possible, group members give a reason for arriving at their idea of what is going on with a patient at a particular time. For example, the group member who felt there were elements of anger and hatred in Margaret's interaction said he was fairly sure he had seen Margaret form her hand into a fist during the interchange with Hugo. He also imitated his idea of her facial expression the one time she looked directly at Hugo. From his demonstration, the glance was much more defiant than scared. Margaret accepted the suggestion that she was experiencing a need for love at the time of her interchange with Hugo. All of the other suggestions were rejected, because she did not feel they really identified how she was feeling.

Following the attempt to identify what the patient is experiencing, the group helps the patient put the behavioral interactions and internal experience together. The sequence of how the patient viewed the situation, what he experienced within himself, and the reasons for his reaction are explored. The patient is urged to try to formulate a relationship. Group members provide feedback. When the group feels the patient has put the situation together in an illogical or incorrect manner, or if the patient is unable to say how external behavior and internal experiences are related, the group provides additional suggestions. Again using the nonverbal behavior that was part of the event, their own experience in similar situations, and their knowledge of the patient, group members suggest possible relationships to the patient. As before, the patient is given ample opportunity to think about the suggestions and is under no pressure to accept any of the suggestions.

In Margaret's group, one suggested relationship was as follows: Margaret accurately perceived Hugo as giving an order. She hid behind the idea of being a little girl so she would not have to tell Hugo he had no right to tell her what to do. Another suggestion was that Margaret so dearly wanted love that she had a negative reaction to anyone who made any kind of demand. She wanted unconditional love, not respect based on her actions. Still another suggestion was that Margaret likes the idea of being a little girl. The more demands she does not meet, the better: Little girls, in her cognitive system, do not meet demands; they avoid them to maintain their status of protected beings. Margaret accepted the last suggestion. At this point, she was able to reverse her previous contention; she liked to maintain the idea that she was really just a little girl.

To help a patient both decide whether the present formulation of the relationship between his behavior and internal experiences is accurate and determine if this is an isolated situation or a regularly occurring pattern, the group helps the patient think about past events in the group and recent events in his interactions outside of the group and treatment center. Both Margaret and the group were able to identify several concrete examples of Margaret not meeting very reasonable demands. This was a typical pattern of behavior.

What Needs to Be Changed?

In this step of the process, the patient is helped to identify what facets of the private self need to be altered. There may be need to change only one facet, or change in many areas may be required. The latter is true for Margaret. For more adequate function, Margaret must develop the idea she is a grown-up person and come to place a high positive value on this idea. She also must find other ways of satisfying her need for love and expressing negative emotions. When there is difficulty in more than one facet, the patient and group members decide which facet will be worked on first. Margaret decided she wanted to stop thinking of herself as a little girl. The necessity for Margaret to learn to meet her need for love was also recognized. It was decided that the therapist and Margaret would work on this area outside the group. Margaret had little idea about how to go about making friends. Thus, the therapist planned to help Margaret develop skills in the area of intimacy. The group was to help Margaret change her ideas about herself.

Learning

After identifying the goal, the patient and the group develop a plan for learning. This includes what the patient will be encouraged to do and what other group members will do. It was decided that group members would insist Margaret take the same responsibilities other group members were asked to take. No assistance would be given unless Margaret truly needed help. The group was to provide feedback to Margaret about how well she was meeting the demands of the situation and compliment her whenever she took responsibility.

To illustrate, at this particular time the group was planning an art exhibit and sale of patient and staff paintings that was to be open to the public. Some of the things Margaret was asked to do were to request permission from the hospital director for use of the front lobby, to go to certain local merchants to ask for donations for door prizes, to assist with hanging the pictures, to be at the front desk from one o'clock until three o'clock each day of the exhibit, and so forth. Although hesitant at first, Margaret soon began to take on responsibilities. The group took no excuses for failure and simply told Margaret she would have to try again. For example, Margaret went to the hospital director's office, became fearful, and left without speaking to the director. The group told her that children act that way, not adults. She pleaded for someone to go with her, but the request was denied. Margaret was sent back to the office. This time she was able to ask for permission. As time went on, Margaret began to see that she could meet normal demands and responsibilities. She also discovered that in so doing other people responded to her differently. Rather than getting less attention and affection, she received more. Margaret slowly began to see herself as an adult.

Follow-Up

Follow-up usually occurs in the discussion at the end of each meeting of the group. At this time the group reviews the events of the session in light of what each group member has been attempting to learn through interacting in the group. Feedback is provided as well as support and encouragement. Once a patient has begun to develop a particular facet of the private self, he is urged to try the newly developed pattern of behavior outside the group setting. The patient then reports back to the group. The group shares his pleasure when he succeeds and encourages him when he experiences difficulty. For example, once Margaret began to take responsibility in the group, group members urged her to behave in a more adult manner on the ward and at home on weekends. With their support, Margaret began to make her own bed, get to meals on time, and volunteer to help clean up the ward kitchen after evening snacks once a week. At home, Margaret began to take care of her own clothes and to prepare Sunday breakfast. One problem Margaret had was to get her parents to recognize that she could take responsibility. They had always treated her as if she was a helpless creature because Margaret had always acted that way. The group helped Margaret tell her parents that she now wanted to act in a more adult manner and to insist that they permit her to behave in such a manner.

The above-outlined steps are repeated over and over again for each patient in the group. Each group member is encouraged both to examine the personal ideas, needs, emotions, and values that influence his behavior and to help other group members do likewise. Self-understanding allows the patient to decide whether there are aspects of himself that he would like to see changed. Working together, group members help each other bring about the desired changes.

SUMMARY

In summary, activities therapy is an action-oriented, doing process designed to help patients acquire the skills they need for living in the wider community. Ideally, they return to full participation in the community with additional knowledge about themselves and the people, objects, events, and institutions that are part of their life situations. The ideal, of course, is not always attained. Some patients are not able to adjust to the community or are able to make only a marginal adjustment. But one could turn that around and state, perhaps more honestly, that the community cannot adjust to or can only marginally adjust to the patient.

Until we have greater understanding of psychosocial dysfunction, activities therapy is presented here as one way of helping people to develop their potential to the greatest possible degree.

SUGGESTED READING

Bernstein, Penny. *Theory and Methods in Dance-Movement Therapy.* Dubuque, Iowa: Kendall/Hunt Publishing Company, 1972.

Burton, Arthur. *Encounter.* San Francisco: Jossey-Boss, 1969.

Diedrich, R., and Dye, C. *Group Procedures: Purposes, Processes and Outcomes.* Boston: Houghton Mifflin Company, 1972.

Fidler, G., *"The Task Oriented Group as a Context for Treatment," American Journal of Occupational Therapy,* 23, 1:43–48 (1969).

Goldberg, Carl. *Encounter: Group Sensitivity Training Experience.* New York: Science House, 1970.

Hammer, Emanuel. *Use of Interpretations in Treatment.* New York: Grune & Stratton, 1968.

Perls, Frederick. *Gestalt Therapy Verbation.* New York: Bantam Books, 1969.

Pesso, Albert. *Movement in Psychotherapy.* New York: New York University Press, 1970.

Rogers, Carl. *Carl Rogers on Encounter Groups.* New York: Harper & Row, 1970.

Yalom, Irvin. *The Theory and Practice of Group Psychotherapy.* New York: Basic Books, 1970.

INDEX